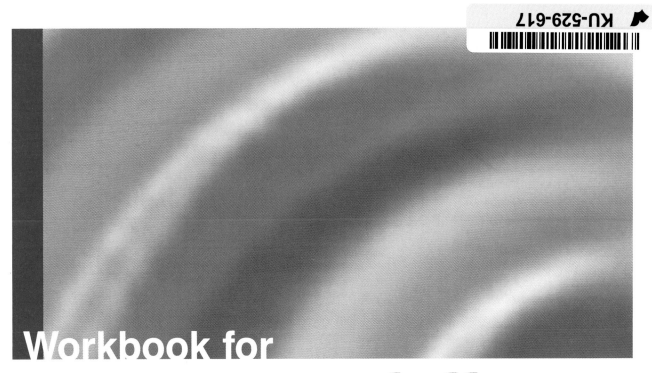

Workbook for

Basic Skills for
Nursing Assistants
in Long-Term Care

Bernie Gorek, RNC, GNP, MA, NHA
Gerontology Consultant
Greeley, Colorado

ELSEVIER
MOSBY

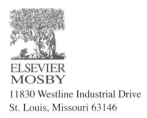

ELSEVIER
MOSBY

11830 Westline Industrial Drive
St. Louis, Missouri 63146

WORKBOOK FOR BASIC SKILLS FOR
NURSING ASSISTANTS IN LONG-TERM CARE

ISBN 0-323-02205-7

International Standard Book Number 0-323-02205-7

Acquisitions Editor: **Susan R. Epstein**
Senior Developmental Editor: **Maria Broeker**
Publishing Services Manager: **John Rogers**
Senior Project Manager: **Kathleen L. Teal**
Senior Designer: **Kathi Gosche**

Printed in the United States of America

Last digit is the print number: 9 8 7 6 5 4 3 2 1

To my aunts, Dolores and Lucille
Thanks for your love and your support

Preface

This workbook is written to be used with Mosby's *Basic Skills for Nursing Assistants in Long-Term Care* textbook, first edition by Sheila A. Sorrentino and Bernie Gorek. The student will not need other resources to complete the exercises in this workbook.

The workbook is designed to help students apply what they have learned in each chapter. Students are encouraged to use the workbook as a study guide. Various types of questions (Matching, Fill in the Blanks, and Multiple Choice) and learning exercises are included in each chapter to help students understand and apply the information in the textbook. The Additional Learning Activities encourage discussion and practical application of the information presented in each chapter. These activities are meant to challenge the student and enhance the learning experience. Procedure Checklists are provided, which correspond with the procedures in each chapter of the *Basic Skills for Nursing Assistants in Long-Term Care* textbook, first edition. These checklists are intended to help students become confident and skilled when performing procedures that affect the quality of care they provide. Answers to the workbook questions are provided in the Instructor's Guide, which accompanies the textbook.

Nursing assistants are important members of the health and nursing teams. Completing the exercises in this workbook will increase each student's knowledge, skills, and confidence. The goal is to prepare students to provide the best possible care and to help them develop pride in the important work they do.

Bernie Gorek

Contents

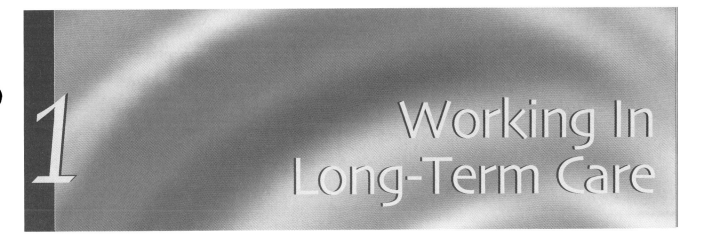

Working In Long-Term Care

OBJECTIVES

The questions and student activities in this chapter will help you meet these objectives.
- Define the key terms listed in Chapter 1
- Describe long-term care facilities and how they are organized
- Identify members of the interdisciplinary health care team and the nursing team
- Describe the nursing service department
- Describe programs that pay for health care
- Explain the purpose and requirements of the Omnibus Budget Reconciliation Act of 1987 (OBRA)
- Explain the roles and responsibilities of nursing assistants
- Explain why a job description is important
- Describe the delegation process and how to use the "five rights of delegation"
- Describe intentional and unintentional torts
- Explain the purpose of informed consent
- Describe your role in recognizing and reporting elder abuse
- Identify good health and personal hygiene practices
- Describe how to look professional
- Describe the qualities and traits of a successful nursing assistant
- Describe ethical behavior on the job
- Explain the aspects of harassment
- Explain why standards are met

Study Questions
Crossword

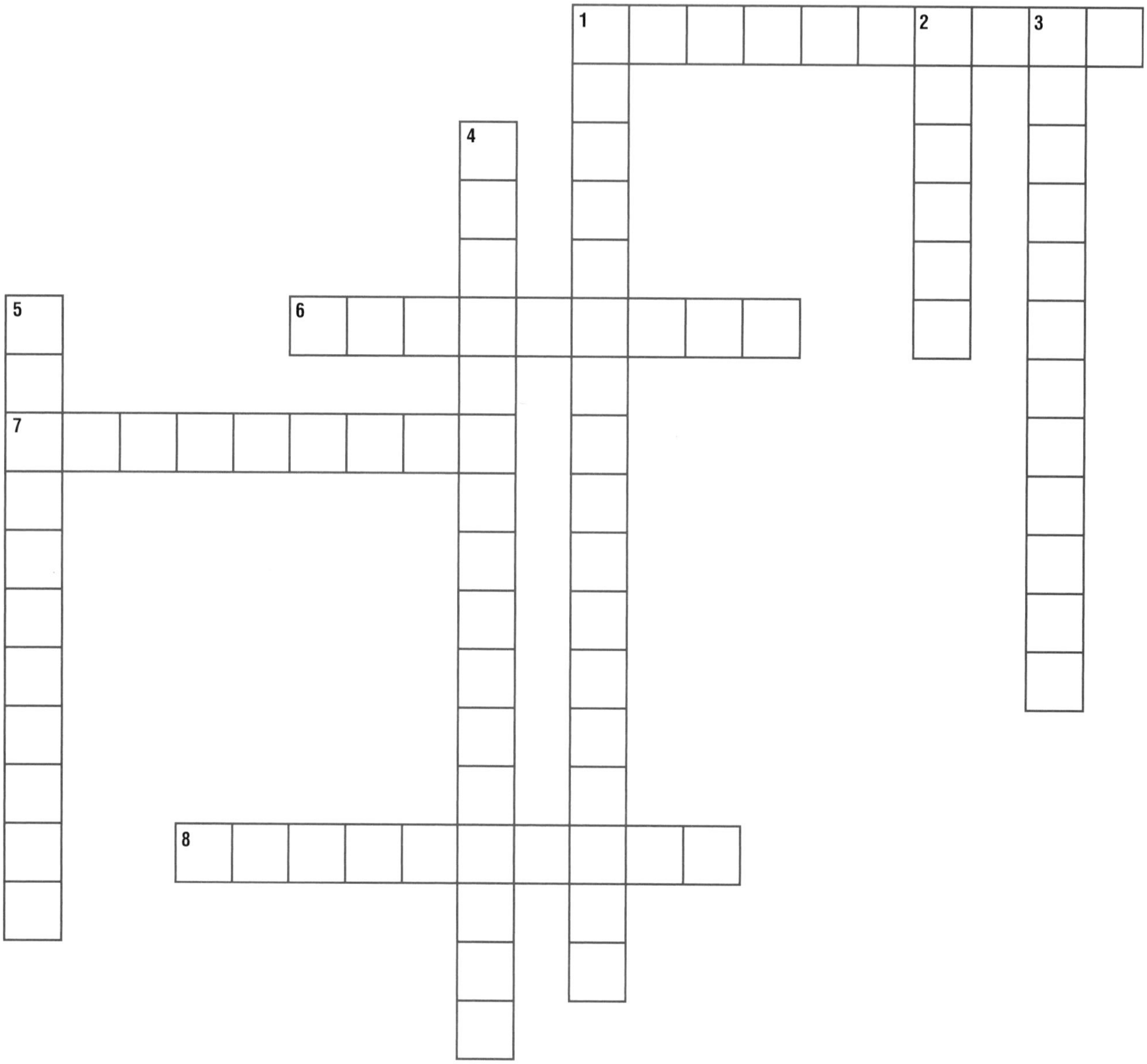

(crossword grid)

Across

1. Fills drug orders written by doctors; monitors and evaluates drug interactions
6. Diagnoses and treats diseases and injuries
7. Assesses and plans for nutritional needs; teaches good nutrition, food selection, and preparation
8. Prevents, diagnoses, and treats foot disorders

Down

1. Assists persons with musculoskeletal problems; focuses on restoring function and preventing disability
2. Assists with spiritual needs
3. Helps residents and families deal with social, emotional, and environmental issues affecting illness and recovery
4. Assists nurses and gives nursing care; supervised by a licensed nurse
5. Tests hearing, prescribes hearing aids, and works with hearing-impaired persons

Matching

Match each term with the correct definition.

1. _____ Trusting others with personal and private information

2. _____ The intentional mistreatment or harm of another person

3. _____ A variety of health workers who work together to provide for the person's total care

4. _____ A nurse who has completed a 1-year nursing program and has passed a licensing test

5. _____ A person who gives basic nursing care under the supervision of a licensed nurse

6. _____ A facility that provides medical, nursing, dietary, recreational, rehabilitative, and social services

7. _____ Making false statements orally

8. _____ A rule of conduct made by a government body

9. _____ A federal law concerned with the quality of life, health, and safety of residents

10. _____ A nurse who has completed a 2-, 3-, or 4-year nursing program and has passed a licensing test

11. _____ An agency or program for persons who are dying

12. _____ Knowledge of what is right conduct and wrong conduct

13. _____ An act that violates a criminal law

14. _____ Unlawful restraint or restriction of a person's movement

A. Hospice

B. Interdisciplinary health care team

C. Abuse

D. Omnibus Budget Reconciliation Act of 1987 (OBRA)

E. Licensed practical nurse (LPN)

F. Registered nurse (RN)

G. Nursing center

H. Crime

I. Nursing assistant

J. Ethics

K. Law

L. Confidentiality

M. Slander

N. False imprisonment

Fill in the Blanks

15. There are many myths about aging and older persons. Identify the myths and facts about aging and older persons in the following statements. Mark M for myth and F for fact.
    A. _____ All old people are the same.
    B. _____ Many older people enjoy a fulfilling sex life.
    C. _____ Older persons are at risk for health problems and disabilities.
    D. _____ Older people are lonely and isolated.
    E. _____ Most older parents see a child at least once a week.
    F. _____ Most older persons live in nursing centers.
    G. _____ Some old people are crabby and rude, as are some people of all ages.

16. Persons who live in long-term care facilities are called _____.

17. Long-term care facilities are designed to meet the needs of older and disabled residents. Describe the following residents you will care for:

    A. Confused and disoriented residents

    _____

    _____

    _____

B. Short-term residents

_____

_____

_____

18. A disability occurring before age 22 is called

_____.

19. List the services provided by nursing centers.

A. _____

B. _____

C. _____

D. _____

E. _____

F. _____

20. A skilled nursing facility (SNF) provides nursing

care for _____

_____

_____

_____.

21. An Alzheimer's unit is designed for _____

_____

_____

_____.

22. _____

provides housing, personal care, support services,

health care, and social services in a home-like setting.

23. Which member of the health care team is responsible for the entire nursing staff and the care given?

_____

_____

24. The goal of the interdisciplinary health care team is

_____.

25. The nursing team involves _____

_____

_____

_____.

26. _____ limit the

amounts paid by insurers, Medicare, and Medicaid.

The amount paid is determined before the person en-

ters the hospital, SNF, or rehabilitation center.

27. OBRA requires each state to have a nursing assistant training and competency evaluation program. How many hours of instruction are required?

_____

How many hours must be supervised practical training?

_____

28. The _____ has

a written test and a skills test.

29. What information about each nursing assistant is contained in the nursing assistant registry?

A. _____

B. _____

C. _____

D. _____

E. _____

F. _____

G. _____

30. Retraining and a new competency evaluation program are required for nursing assistants who have not worked for _____.

31. To protect persons from harm, you must understand:

   A. _____

   B. _____

   C. _____

32. _____ is a list of responsibilities and functions the center expects you to perform.

33. You should not take a job that requires you to:

   A. _____

   B. _____

   C. _____

34. An RN can delegate tasks to you. A task is

_____

_____.

35. You perform a task delegated to you by the RN. Who is legally responsible for the delegated task?

_____

36. _____ and _____ state the tasks that nurses can delegate to you.

37. List "the five rights of delegation."

   A. _____

   B. _____

   C. _____

   D. _____

   E. _____

38. When you agree to perform a delegated task, you must _____.

39. To be prejudiced or biased means _____ _____ _____.

40. You do not act in a reasonable or careful manner. As a result a person is harmed. This is _____ _____.

41. Malpractice is _____ _____.

42. Which staff members are allowed to see, touch, or examine a person's body?

_____

_____

_____

43. HIPAA protects the privacy and security of a person's health information. Protected health information refers to _____ _____ _____.

44. Consent is informed when _____ _____ _____.

45. Define the following forms of elder abuse:

    A. Physical abuse

    _____

    _____

    _____

    _____

    B. Involuntary seclusion

    _____

    _____

    _____

46. OBRA does not allow nursing centers to employ persons who were convicted of _____

    _____

    _____.

47. Employers want employees who:

    A. _____

    B. _____

    C. _____

    D. _____

48. Why should you avoid gossip in the work place?

    _____

    _____

49. Why is it important to keep personal matters out of the work place?

    _____

    _____

    _____

50. Plan your work to _____

    _____ and to

    _____.

51. You feel that a co-worker is sexually harassing you. What should you do?

    _____

    _____

52. Why are surveys done in nursing centers?

    _____

    _____

    _____

Circle the BEST Answer

53. The study of the aging process is
    A. Geriatrics
    B. Gerontology
    C. Aging science
    D. Delegation

54. The nursing team
    A. Focuses on tasks and jobs
    B. Involves the individuals who provide nursing care
    C. Involves a primary nurse who is responsible for the resident's total care
    D. Involves doctors, nurses, and social workers

55. Which is a federal health insurance program for persons 65 years of age and older and for some younger people with disabilities?
    A. Private insurance
    B. Medicare
    C. Medicaid
    D. Prospective payment

56. Managed care
    A. Is a health insurance plan sponsored by the federal government
    B. Is a nursing care pattern
    C. Deals with health care delivery and payment
    D. Is required by OBRA

57. The nursing assistant registry is
    A. A skills evaluation
    B. An official record of persons who have completed a state-approved training and competency evaluation program
    C. A list of rules and responsibilities for nursing assistants
    D. A procedure book

58. Nursing assistants
    A. Function under the supervision of RNs or LPNs/LVNs
    B. Decide what should or should *not* be done for a person
    C. Supervise other nursing assistants
    D. Take telephone orders from the doctor

59. You can refuse to do a delegated task for all of the following reasons, *except*
    A. The task is not in your job description.
    B. You do not know how to use the equipment.
    C. You are busy and the task is unpleasant.
    D. The nurse's directions are unclear.

60. You agree to perform a task; therefore you
    A. Are responsible for your own actions
    B. Can perform the task as soon as you have time
    C. Must report what you did and your observations to the doctor
    D. Can delegate the task to another nursing assistant if you do not have time to perform it yourself

61. You suspect a person you are caring for is being abused. You must
    A. Report your observations to the nurse.
    B. Call the police.
    C. Tell a co-worker.
    D. Tell the person's doctor.

62. Threatening a person with punishment is
    A. Physical abuse
    B. Neglect
    C. Mental abuse
    D. Sexual abuse

63. Which statement signals a bad attitude?
    A. "Thank you for your help."
    B. "Can I help you with that?"
    C. "Is there anything else I can do?"
    D. "I can't. I'm too busy."

64. To keep personal matters out of the work place, you should
    A. Carry your cell phone with you and have it turned on at all times.
    B. Discuss your personal problems with your co-workers.
    C. Use center copy machines to copy recipes.
    D. Make doctors appointments for your days off.

65. Your role in the survey process involves
    A. Providing quality care
    B. Reviewing residents' medical records
    C. Interviewing members of the survey team
    D. Talking to family members about the survey process

Additional Learning Activities

1. Look in the yellow pages of the telephone book and list the health care agencies in your community along with the services they provide.

2. Write about an experience you or a family member had with a health care agency. Answer these questions:

   A. What was the purpose of the contact?

   B. What type of agency was it?

   C. What members of the health care team were involved?

   D. What were the roles of each member of the team?

3. Provide the following information about RNs, LPNs/LVNs, and assistive personnel:

    A. Education requirements

    B. Licensure requirements

    C. Roles and responsibilities

4. Look at your health insurance policy. Do you know which services are covered and which are not? Does your policy limit where you can go for health care? Explain.

5. Read the rules of conduct for nursing assistants.

    A. Write down ways to apply these rules in a job setting.

    B. Discuss the importance of these rules with your classmates.

6. You are asked to do a task that you feel is unsafe.

    A. How would you handle the situation?

    B. What could you say?

    C. Which health team member would you talk to about your concerns?

7. Are there any job functions that you are opposed to doing for moral or religious reasons? Explain.

    A. How will you advise your employer of your concerns?

8. Use the yellow pages of the phone book or the internet to look up agencies in your community that deal with abuse.

    A. List the services each agency provides.

9. You are preparing for a job interview. How will you make a good impression?

How will you show the employer that you have what he or she is looking for in these areas?

A. Hygiene measures

B. Professional appearance

C. Skills and training

D. Values and attitude

10. You have succeeded in getting the job you want. Now, it is important to keep your job. How will you make sure that:

A. You have dependable transportation?

B You have childcare, if needed?

C. You get to work on time?

D. You are available to work at the times you are scheduled?

E. You stay healthy so you can function at your best?

2 Communication and Interpersonal Skills

OBJECTIVES

The questions and student activities in this chapter will help you meet these objectives.
- Define the key terms listed in Chapter 2
- Explain why health team members need to communicate
- Describe the rules for good communication
- Explain the purpose, parts, and information found in the medical record
- Describe the legal and ethical aspects of medical records
- Describe the rules for answering phones
- Explain how to deal with conflict
- Identify the parts that make up the whole person
- Explain Abraham Maslow's theory of basic needs
- Explain how culture and religion influence health and illness
- Describe how to use verbal and nonverbal communication
- Explain the methods and barriers to good communication
- Explain how to communicate with persons with disabilities
- Explain why families and visitors are important to the person

Study Questions
Matching

Match each term with the correct definition.

1. _____ Messages sent through facial expressions, gestures, posture, hand and body movements, gait, eye contact, and appearance

2. _____ The exchange of information

3. _____ Something necessary or desired for maintaining life and mental well-being

4. _____ Spiritual beliefs, needs, and practices

5. _____ The inability to speak

6. _____ A written account of a person's condition and response to treatment and care; chart

7. _____ Communication that uses written or spoken words

8. _____ A lost, absent, or impaired physical or mental function

9. _____ The characteristics of a group of people passed from one generation to the next

10. _____ Difficulty receiving information

A. Medical record

B. Need

C. Disability

D. Verbal communication

E. Religion

F. Aphasia

G. Culture

H. Communication

I. Receptive aphasia

J. Body language

Fill in the Blanks

11. The medical record is _____

    and is a _____ document.

12. If you have access to the medical record you must

    _____

    _____.

13. List and briefly describe the parts of the medical record that relate to your work?

    A. _____

    _____

    _____

    B. _____

    _____

    _____

    C. _____

    _____

    _____

14. The Omnibus Budget Reconciliation Act of 1987 (OBRA) requires that the health team be involved in planning the person's care. Planning involves

    _____.

15. The person's comprehensive care plan identifies the person's:

    A. _____

    B. _____

    C. _____

    D. _____

16. What information should you write down when taking a phone message?

    A. _____

    B. _____

    C. _____

17. You have answered the phone at the nurses' station. The caller asks you for confidential information about a resident. What should you do?

    _____

    _____

18. What can happen if you do not work out conflict in the workplace?

    _____

    _____

19. List the six steps in the problem-solving process.

    A. _____

    B. _____

    C. _____

    D. _____

    E. _____

    F. _____

20. The _____ is the most important person in the center.

21. The whole person has _____, _____, _____, and _____ parts.

22. _____ needs are needed to survive.

23. Safety and security needs relate to _____

_____

_____.

24. Culture affects health care beliefs and practices.

Some _____ believe that

illness is caused when hot and cold are not in balance.

Some _____ add

herbs to drinks and enemas to treat stomach acidity.

25. The _____ reflects

the person's culture and religion.

26. Follow these rules for verbal communication:

A. _____

B. _____

C. _____

D. _____

E. _____

F. _____

G. _____

H. _____

27. _____ communication

does not use words.

28. Touch is an important form of communication. Touch

conveys _____

_____

_____

_____.

29. To use touch, follow _____

_____.

30. Touch practices vary among cultures. In

_____, men

do not shake hands with women.

31. Certain methods help communication.

_____ means

to focus on verbal and nonverbal communication.

You use sight, hearing, touch, and smell.

32. You are caring for Mr. Adams. You ask, "Mr. Adams,

when would you like your bath?" This is a

_____.

33. What is the purpose of an open-ended question?

_____

_____

34. _____ is a

useful communication method when the person is

upset and needs to gain control.

35. Why is using unfamiliar language a communication
barrier?

_____

_____

_____

36. _____ make

the person feel that you do not care about his or her

concerns, feelings, and fears.

37. Ms. Jensen cannot speak or hear. How will you communicate with her?

_____

_____

_____

38. List five symptoms of hearing loss.

A. _____

B. _____

C. _____

D. _____

E. _____

39. Deafness is _____

_____

_____.

40. Why does the hearing-impaired person hear better with a hearing aid?

_____

_____

41. Ms. Gray tells you that her hearing aid is *not* working. What measures should you try?

A. _____

B. _____

C. _____

D. _____

42. _____ is a

writing system that uses raised dots.

43. _____ or

_____ are used

by blind persons worldwide to move about.

44. Aphasia is the inability to speak. _____

is difficulty expressing or sending out thoughts.

_____ relates to difficulty

receiving information.

45. When communicating with a person who is comatose, you must assume that the person

_____

_____.

46. Explain how the presence of family and friends might affect the person's recovery and quality of life.

_____

_____

_____

_____

47. Mr. Braun has visitors. You must assist him onto the bedpan. What should you do?

_____

_____

Circle the BEST Answer

48. For good communication, do all of the following *except*
    A. Use familiar words.
    B. Be brief and concise.
    C. Give unneeded information.
    D. Give information in a logical and orderly manner.

49. Vertigo means
    A. Deafness
    B. Ringing in the ears
    C. Mild hearing loss
    D. Dizziness

50. An infection in the middle ear is called
    A. Tinnitus
    B. Tympanic
    C. Otitis media
    D. Meniere's disease

51. When communicating with the speech-impaired person, you should
    A. Write everything on white paper.
    B. Ask the person to repeat or rephrase statements if necessary.
    C. Pretend you understand to avoid embarrassment.
    D. Talk loudly.

52. Ms. Lewis is hearing impaired. She wears hearing aids in both ears. To communicate with her, you should do all of the following *except*
    A. Stand above her and look down at her face.
    B. Face her when speaking.
    C. Make sure she is wearing her hearing aids and they are on and working.
    D. Speak clearly, distinctly, and slowly.

53. The sclera of the eye is
    A. The second layer, which contains the blood vessels
    B. The white of the eye, the outer layer
    C. The inner layer, which contains the optic nerve
    D. The chamber filled with aqueous humor

54. To communicate with a blind person, do all of the following *except*
    A. Face the person.
    B. Insist on helping the person for the person's safety.
    C. Use a normal tone of voice.
    D. Keep the signal light within the person's reach.

Additional Learning Activities

1. List some ways that knowing about a person's cultural and religious practices can help you give better care.

2. Do you have cultural or religious beliefs that are important to you? Explain.

    A. How do these beliefs influence your health practices?

3. Practice answering the telephone and taking a message. You can do this with a classmate or with a family member.

    A. How would you answer the telephone in a professional, courteous manner?

B. What information should you get when taking a message?

C. What would you do before putting a person on hold?

4. Read the following vignette involving conflict in the workplace; then answer the questions at the end of the vignette.

    You are assigned to care for Mrs. Angie Gomez. When you return from your lunch break, Mrs. Gomez's signal light is on. When you answer her signal light, Mrs. Gomez tells you that her light has been on for 25 minutes. She also tells you that another nursing assistant walked into her room and told Mrs. Gomez that she would have to wait until you returned from lunch.

A. How would you feel?

B. How might Mr. Brian's hearing and vision impairment affect his ability to care for himself?

B. What might you say to Mrs. Gomez?

C. How might Mr. Brian's hearing and vision impairments affect his social life?

C. With whom would you discuss the situation?

D. How can you promote Mr. Brian's safety?

D. Where would you discuss the situation?

E. What measures do you need to practice when caring for Mr. Brian's eyeglasses and hearing aids?

E. What steps would you take to solve the problem?

F. What measures might help you communicate effectively with Mr. Brian?

5. Read the vignette and answer the questions that follow.

Mr. Brian is a 78-year-old nursing center resident. He has a doctoral degree in mathematics. He was the head of the mathematics department at the state university. He has poor vision and is hearing impaired. He wears hearing aids in both ears.

A. What measures might be needed for effective communication with Mr. Brian?

6. Simulate hearing loss by using earplugs in both ears. Then participate in these activities:

A. Watch a movie on TV.

B. Call a friend on the telephone.

C. Go to the grocery store and shop for food items. ***(Do not drive a car with earplugs in place.)***

    (1) How did you feel when performing these routine activities with a hearing impairment?

    (2) Were you ever frustrated?

    (3) Did you feel others were frustrated or impatient with you?

    (4) Did you feel left out?

    (5) How will your experience affect the care you provide?

7. Simulate vision impairment by wearing a pair of eyeglasses with crushed cellophane or petroleum jelly over the lenses. Then try to perform the following activities:
A. Write a letter.
B. Do a load of laundry.
C. Watch a movie on TV.
D. Prepare a simple snack.

    (1) How did your vision impairment affect your ability to perform these simple activities?

    (2) Did you feel uncertain or unsafe when performing any of the activities?

    (3) How will your experience affect the care you provide?

3 Preventing Infection

OBJECTIVES

The questions and student activities in this chapter will help you meet these objectives.
- Define the key terms listed in Chapter 3
- Identify what microbes need to live and grow
- List the signs and symptoms of infection
- Explain the chain of infection
- Describe the changes in the immune system that occur with aging
- Describe aseptic practices
- Explain how to care for equipment and supplies
- Explain Standard Precautions and Transmission-Based Precautions and the Bloodborne Pathogen Standard
- Perform the procedures described in Chapter 3

Study Questions

Crossword

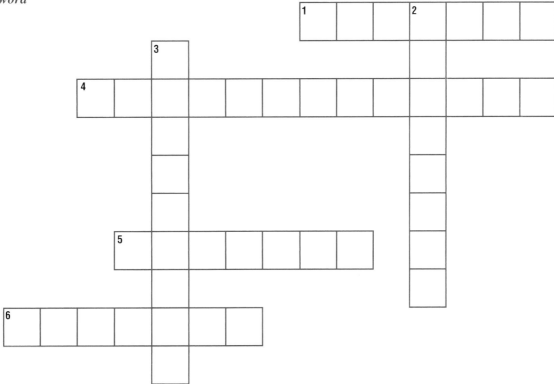

Across

1. Being free of disease-producing microbes
4. The process of becoming unclean
5. The absence of all microbes
6. A microorganism

Down

2. A microbe that is harmful and can cause infection
3. A disease resulting from the invasion and growth of microbes in the body

Matching

Match each term with the correct definition.

1. _____ Items contaminated with blood, body fluids, secretions, and excretions and that may be harmful to others

2. _____ A human or animal that is a reservoir for microbes but does not have signs and symptoms of infection

3. _____ A disease caused by pathogens that spread easily; a contagious disease

4. _____ Medical asepsis

5. _____ The process of destroying pathogens

6. _____ A small living plant or animal seen only with a microscope

7. _____ A microbe that does not usually cause an infection

8. _____ The process of destroying all microbes

9. _____ Methods to prevent the spread of infection

A. Carrier

B. Microorganism

C. Sterilization

D. Biohazardous waste

E. Disinfection

F. Clean technique

G. Non-pathogen

H. Communicable disease

I. Infection control

Fill in the Blanks

10. Microbes need a _____ to live and grow.

11. A _____ infection is in a body part.

A _____ infection involves the whole body.

12. To leave the reservoir, the pathogen needs a _____.

13. List the portals of exit and portals of entry used by pathogens.

A. _____

B. _____

C. _____

D. _____

E. _____

F. _____

14. Medical asepsis is the practices used to:

A. _____

_____

B. _____

_____

15. _____ break the chain of infection.

16. The _____ protects the body from disease and infection.

17. Why are older persons at risk for infections?

_____

_____

_____

18. Pneumonia is _____.

19. _____ is

    the easiest and most important way to prevent the

    spread of infection.

20. Acquired immunodeficiency syndrome (AIDS) is

    caused by the _____

    _____

    _____.

21. Human immunodeficiency virus (HIV) is transmitted
    mainly by:

    A. _____

    B. _____

    C. _____

    D. _____

22. Sexually transmitted diseases (STDs) are spread by

    _____

    _____

    _____.

23. _____ is a

    skin disorder in which the female mite burrows into

    the skin and lays eggs.

24. Drug resistant organisms are _____

    _____

    _____.

25. List the two main causes of drug resistant organisms.

    A. _____

    B. _____

26. To prevent the spread of infection, you must wash
    your hands with soap and water:

    A. _____

    _____

    B. _____

    _____

    C. _____

    _____

27. Use _____ to

    decontaminate your hands if they are not visibly soiled.

28. When should you wear a gown?

    _____

    _____

    _____

29. Used syringes and needles, scalpel blades, and other

    sharp items are placed in _____

    _____.

30. How many paper towels should you use to turn off
    faucets after hand washing?

    _____

31. Cleaning does the following:

    A. _____

    _____

    B. _____

    _____

32. You are cleaning a contaminated surface. You must

    clean _____

    from your body.

33. Isolation Precautions are based on

    _____ and _____.

34. _____ reduce

    the risk of spreading pathogens and known and un-

    known infections. They are used for all persons.

35. Some infections require Transmission-Based Precau-

    tions. The type used depends on _____

    _____.

36. Ms. Gomez is on Transmission-Based Precautions.
    What information do you need from the nurse and the
    care plan before providing care?

    A. _____

    B. _____

    C. _____

37. Contact Precautions are used for known or suspected
    infections involving microbes transmitted by:

    A. _____

       _____

    B. _____

       _____

38. Wear gloves whenever contact with

    _____,

    _____,

    _____,

    _____,

    _____, and

    _____ is likely.

39. Gloves are easier to put on when your hands are

    _____.

40. Remove and discard _____,

    _____, or

    _____ gloves at once.

41. You notice an itchy rash on your hands after you re-
    move your gloves. What should you do?

    _____

    _____

42. Masks prevent the spread of microbes from the

    _____.

43. When removing a mask, only touch the

    _____.

    The front of the mask is _____.

44. _____ protect

    your eyes, mouth, and nose from splashing or spraying

    of blood, body fluids, secretions, or excretions.

45. The person's _____,

    _____, and

    _____ needs

    are often unmet when Isolation Precautions are used.

46. The _____

    protects workers from exposure to the AIDS virus

    (HIV) and the hepatitis virus.

47. When are work surfaces decontaminated?

    A. _____

    B. _____

    C. _____

    D. _____

48. What precautions does Occupational Safety and Health Administration (OSHA) require for contaminated laundry?

    A. _____

    _____

    B. _____

    _____

    C. _____

    _____

    D. _____

    _____

    E. _____

    _____

49. An exposure incident is _____

    _____

    _____.

50. _____ means

    piercing the mucous membranes or the skin barrier.

51. The _____ is

    the person whose blood or body fluids are the source

    of an exposure incident.

Circle the BEST Answer

52. The most important measure to prevent the spread of infection is
    A. Sterilization of equipment
    B. Hand hygiene
    C. Surgical asepsis
    D. Isolation precautions

53. The environment where microbes live and grow is the
    A. Infection
    B. Portal of entry
    C. Reservoir or host
    D. Source

54. Tuberculosis is spread by
    A. Soiled dressings
    B. Airborne droplets
    C. Feces
    D. Contaminated drinking water

55. Hepatitis is
    A. A urinary bladder infection
    B. An inflammation of the lungs
    C. A local infection
    D. An inflammation of the liver

56. Hepatitis A is spread by
    A. The fecal-oral route
    B. Sharing needles
    C. Contaminated blood products
    D. Inhaling cocaine through contaminated straws

57. The infestation of the body with lice is
    A. Pediculosis capitis
    B. Body pediculosis
    C. Pediculosis corporis
    D. Pediculosis pubis

58. You help prevent the chain of infection by all of the following *except*
    A. Washing your hands after urinating
    B. Washing your hands before and after handling food
    C. Covering your nose and mouth when coughing
    D. Washing your hands every 2 hours

59. To wash your hands, do the following:
    A. Use very hot running water.
    B. Stand with your body touching the sink.
    C. Keep your hands and forearms higher than your elbows.
    D. Clean your fingernails by rubbing them against your palms. Use a nail file or an orange stick to clean under the nails.

60. Which statement about wearing gloves is *incorrect?*
    A. Wear gloves when touching blood, body fluids, secretions, and excretions.
    B. Wear the same gloves for all tasks and procedures performed on the same person.
    C. Remove gloves promptly after use.
    D. Decontaminate your hands at once after removing gloves.

61. All non-pathogens and pathogens are destroyed by
    A. Disinfection
    B. Cleaning
    C. Sterilization
    D. Hand washing

62. Disposable gloves are worn when using chemical disinfectants.
    A. True
    B. False

63. You help prevent the spread of infection by
    A. Cleaning toward your body
    B. Using leak-proof plastic bags for soiled linens
    C. Holding equipment and linens against your uniform
    D. Cleaning from the dirtiest area to the cleanest area

64. Isolation precautions involve
    A. Wearing gloves, gowns, and a mask
    B. Special procedures for removing trash from the room
    C. Special measures to collect specimens
    D. All of the above

65. Protective gowns
    A. Protect against splashes and sprays
    B. Open in the front
    C. Are used more than once
    D. Are clean on the outside

66. A wet gown is contaminated.
    A. True
    B. False

67. Which of the following is *not* a sign or symptom of infection?
    A. Fever
    B. Increased appetite
    C. Pain and tenderness
    D. Redness and swelling

68. Which of the following is an aseptic measure?
    A. Taking equipment from one person's room to another
    B. Holding equipment and linen close to your uniform
    C. Covering your nose and mouth when coughing or sneezing
    D. Sitting on a resident's bed when talking to him or her

69. You can receive the hepatis B vaccination within 10 working days of being hired. The center pays for it.
    A. True
    B. False

Additional Learning Activities

1. List the measures you practice in your personal life to prevent infection.

2. List the special care needs of persons on Transmission-Based Precautions. How can you help meet their needs?

3. Carefully review the procedures in Chapter 3.
   A. Practice the procedures for hand washing, removing gloves, wearing a mask, donning and removing a gown, and double bagging.

      (1) Use the procedure checklists provided on pages 124-127 as a guide.

OBJECTIVES

The questions and student activities in this chapter will help you meet these objectives.
- Define the key terms listed in Chapter 4
- Describe how aging and common health problems affect the musculoskeletal system
- Describe accident risk factors
- Explain how to use good body mechanics
- Explain how to accurately identify a person before giving care
- Explain how to use the call system
- Describe how to prevent falls, burns, poisoning, and equipment accidents
- Explain how to handle hazardous substances
- Identify the sources and equipment used in oxygen therapy
- Describe safety measures for oxygen use and fire prevention
- Explain what to do during a fire
- Give examples of natural and human-made disasters
- Explain how to protect yourself from workplace violence
- Describe your role in risk management
- Perform the procedures described in Chapter 4

Study Questions

Matching

Match each term with the correct definition.

1. _____ The way the head, trunk, arms, and legs are aligned with one another; posture

2. _____ The area on which an object rests

3. _____ A state of being unaware of one's surroundings and being unable to react or respond to people, places, or things

4. _____ Using the body in an efficient and careful way

5. _____ Any event that has or could harm a resident, staff member, or visitor

6. _____ Any chemical in the workplace that can cause harm

7. _____ Violent acts directed toward persons at work or while on duty

A. Base of support

B. Coma

C. Workplace violence

D. Body alignment

E. Hazardous substance

F. Incident

G. Body mechanics

Fill in the Blanks

8. The health team must keep residents safe. What is the goal?

   _____

   _____

9. List seven factors that increase a person's risk of injury.

   A. _____

   B. _____

   C. _____

   D. _____

   E. _____

   F. _____

   G. _____

10. _____,

    _____,

    and _____ result

    when the body is not used or positioned properly.

11. How should you stand for a wider base of support and more balance?

    _____

12. For good body mechanics, bend your

    _____ and

    _____ to lift a heavy

    object. Do not _____

    _____.

13. Holding objects away from your body places strain

    on _____

    _____.

14. Ergonomics is _____

    _____

    _____.

15. What is the goal of ergonomics?

    _____

    _____

16. _____

    involve injuries to the muscles, tendons, ligaments,

    joints, cartilage, and nervous system.

17. You must give the right care to the right person. To identify the person before giving care, you must:

    A. _____

       _____

       _____

    B. _____

       _____

       _____

       _____

18. Ms. Green lives at Pine Ridge Nursing Center. She chooses not to wear an identification (ID) bracelet. How can you safely identify her before giving care?

    _____

    _____

19. Always keep the signal light _____

    _____.

20. Mr. Jamison is paralyzed on his right. On which side should you place his signal light?

    _____

21. When do most falls occur?

22. List three safety measures to help prevent falls in bathrooms.

A.

B.

C.

23. The _____ and _____ tell you when to raise bed rails.

24. Bed rails present hazards. Entrapment is a risk.

Entrapment means that _____

25. Bed rails cannot be used unless they are needed to

26. The bed is in the _____ position, except when giving bedside care.

27. Why is a safety check made of the resident's room after visitors leave?

28. Casters on wheelchairs must point _____.

This keeps the wheelchair

29. How many workers are needed for a safe stretcher transfer?

30. You are assisting Ms. Bennet to walk. She starts to fall. What should you do?

31. What are the purposes of hand rails and grab bars?

32. Bed legs have wheels. When are bed wheels locked?

33. You must always _____ on beds, wheelchairs, and stretchers before you transfer a person.

34. List four common causes of burns.

A.

B.

C.

D.

35. Heat and cold applications can cause _____

_____.

36. List five reasons a doctor might order heat applications.

 A. _____

 B. _____

 C. _____

 D. _____

 E. _____

37. Dilate means to _____

_____.

38. Why are lower temperatures used for moist heat applications than for dry heat applications?

_____

_____

_____

39. Cold applications are used to:

 A. _____

 B. _____

 C. _____

40. _____ means to

 narrow.

41. Complications from cold applications include:

 A. _____

 B. _____

 C. _____

42. Before applying heat or cold, what information do you need from the nurse and the care plan?

 A. _____

 B. _____

 C. _____

 D. _____

 E. _____

 F. _____

 G. _____

43. You have applied a warm compress to Mr. Day's right leg. How often do you need to observe his skin at the application site?

_____

44. You have applied a dry cold application to Ms.

 Evan's left forearm. You should secure the application

 in place with _____,

 _____, or

 _____. Do not

 use _____.

45. When is equipment unsafe?

 A. _____

 B. _____

 C. _____

46. Frayed cords and overloaded electrical outlets can

 cause _____ and

 _____.

47. Mr. Flynn brings a reading lamp from home. What should you do?

_____

_____

48. Why are electrical items turned off before they are unplugged?

_____

_____

49. The _____

requires that agencies report equipment-related

illnesses, injuries, and deaths.

50. Exposure to hazardous substances can occur in the workplace. List six hazardous substances you might be exposed to in the workplace.

A. _____

B. _____

C. _____

D. _____

E. _____

F. _____

51. Hazardous substance containers need warning labels. What should you do if a warning label is removed or damaged?

_____

_____

52. Every hazardous substance has a material safety data sheet (MSDS). When must you check the MSDS?

_____

_____

53. Oxygen is supplied in the following ways:

A. _____

B. _____

C. _____

D. _____

54. Oxygen is treated as a _____.

55. Which health team members are responsible for

starting and maintaining oxygen therapy?

_____

_____

56. Describe the following devices used to give oxygen.

A. Nasal cannula

_____

_____

_____

B. Simple mask

_____

_____

_____

57. The flow rate is _____

_____.

58. Mr. Perry is receiving oxygen by nasal cannula. The nurse tells you that the flow rate is 3 liters per minute. When you get him up to the bathroom, you notice that the flow rate is 4 liters per minute. What should you do?

_____

59. Why is oxygen often humidified?

_____

_____

_____

60. Ms. Larken is receiving oxygen by simple mask at 2 liters per minute. You walk by her room and notice that her son is sitting next to her bed and is smoking. What should you do?

_____

_____

61. List the three things needed for a fire.

    A. _____

    B. _____

    C. _____

62. The word RACE will help you remember what to do first if a fire occurs. What do the letters *R-A-C-E* stand for?

    A. _____

    B. _____

    C. _____

    D. _____

63. You are using a fire extinguisher. After you remove

    the safety pin, you should direct the hose

    _____.

64. A disaster is _____

    _____

    _____.

65. Often bomb threats are made by phone. If a caller

    makes a bomb threat, you must _____

    _____

    _____.

66. Why are nurses and nursing assistants at risk for workplace violence?

    _____

    _____

67. The goal of violence prevention programs is to

    _____

    _____.

68. Risk management involves _____

    _____

    _____.

69. You must report accidents and errors at once. What do accidents and errors include?

    A. _____

    B. _____

    C. _____

    D. _____

    E. _____

70. List seven signs and symptoms that may occur with a fracture.

    A. _____

    B. _____

    C. _____

    D. _____

    E. _____

    F. _____

    G. _____

71. A _____ is an injury

    to a ligament. The ligament is torn or stretched.

Circle the BEST Answer

72. Which statement about bed rails is *false?*
    A. Bed rails prevent persons from getting out of bed.
    B. Bed rails are needed for all nursing center residents.
    C. A person can get caught or entangled in bed rails.
    D. Bed rails can cause serious injury and death.

73. Which action will help prevent equipment accidents?
    A. Turning off equipment before unplugging it
    B. Using electrical items near water
    C. Running electrical cords under rugs
    D. Trying to repair broken items yourself

74. Which practice is *unsafe* when using electric beds?
    A. Plugging the power cord into an extension cord
    B. Checking the power cord for damage or fraying
    C. Making sure the bed moves up and down freely
    D. Reporting any unusual sounds or odors

75. Which is a wheelchair safety measure?
    A. Letting the person's feet drag on the floor when the chair is moving
    B. Pulling the chair backwards
    C. Letting the person stand on the footrests when repositioning
    D. Locking both wheels before you transfer a person to or from the wheelchair

76. You find a bottle of liquid in the tub room without a label. You should
    A. Open it to see what is inside.
    B. Leave the container and get the nurse.
    C. Take the container to the nurse and explain the problem.
    D. Ask a co-worker what is in the container.

77. Special safety precautions are practiced where oxygen is used and stored.
    A. True
    B. False

78. The first thing you must do when a fire occurs is to
    A. Pull the fire alarm.
    B. Rescue persons in immediate danger.
    C. Get the fire extinguisher.
    D. Turn off electrical equipment.

79. Which is a fire prevention measure?
    A. Emptying ashtrays into wastebaskets
    B. Smoking in resident rooms
    C. Using a lighter instead of matches to light cigarettes when the person is receiving oxygen
    D. Storing flammable liquids in their original containers

80. When dealing with an agitated or aggressive person, you should
    A. Use touch to calm the person.
    B. Keep your hands free.
    C. Tell the person to calm down.
    D. Stand close to the person.

81. Accidents and errors in care are reported only if someone is injured.
    A. True
    B. False

82. The point at which two or more bones meets is a
    A. Ligament
    B. Joint
    C. Irregular bone
    D. Skeletal muscle

83. This type of muscle can be consciously controlled.
    A. Voluntary muscle
    B. Cardiac muscle
    C. Involuntary muscle
    D. Automatic muscles

84. As a person ages, muscle atrophy and decrease in strength occur.
    A. True
    B. False

85. Arthritis means
    A. Degenerative joint disease
    B. Joint stiffness
    C. Joint inflammation
    D. Hip pain

86. With osteoporosis
    A. There is inflammation of the long bones
    B. Joints are warm and swollen
    C. Joints are stiff and painful
    D. Bones become porous and brittle

87. Which is *not* a factor increasing the risk for falls?
    A. A history of falls
    B. Shoes that fit poorly
    C. Answering signal lights promptly
    D. Low blood pressure

88. Improper use of wheelchairs, walkers, canes, and crutches increases the risk for falls.
    A. True
    B. False

Additional Learning Activities

1. Carefully review the safety measures to prevent falls.

   A. List the safety measures you practice in your home to prevent falls.

   B. List the safety measures you practice in your work setting to prevent falls.

2. Do you have a fire safety plan in your home? Explain.

   A. If you do not already have one, develop an evacuation plan for your home. Make sure that there are at least two possible exits from each room. Have regular fire drills with your family.

3. Review the rules for good body mechanics.

   A. Do you practice these rules in your daily activities? Explain.

   B. Do you practice these rules in your work activities? Explain.

   C. How can you change how you move, lift, and work to decrease your risk for injury?

4. Under the supervision of your instructor:

   A. Use the procedure checklist on page 128 to review and practice the procedure for helping the falling person.

   B. Use the procedure checklist on page 130 to review and practice the procedure for using a fire extinguisher.

5 Basic Emergency Care

OBJECTIVES

The questions and student activities in this chapter will help you meet these objectives.
- Define the key terms listed in Chapter 5
- Describe the general rules of emergency care
- Identify the signs of cardiac arrest and obstructed airway
- Describe the signs, symptoms, and emergency care for hemorrhage
- Identify the signs, symptoms, and emergency care for shock
- Describe the types of seizures and how to care for a person during a seizure
- Identify the common causes and emergency care for fainting
- Identify the emergency care for vomiting and aspiration
- Describe the signs, symptoms, and emergency care for stroke
- Perform the procedures described in Chapter 5

Study Questions

Matching

Match each term with the correct definition.

1. _____ The heart and breathing stop suddenly and without warning

2. _____ Violent and sudden contractions or tremors of muscle groups

3. _____ The sudden loss of consciousness as a result of an inadequate blood supply to the brain; syncope

4. _____ The excessive loss of blood in a short period of time

5. _____ Breathing fluid or an object into the lungs

6. _____ A seizure

7. _____ Results when organs and tissues do not get enough oxygen

A. Convulsion

B. Hemorrhage

C. Cardiac arrest

D. Seizure

E. Fainting

F. Shock

G. Aspiration

Fill in the Blanks

8. When the heart and breathing stop, the person is

_____.

9. What are the three major signs of cardiac arrest?

A. _____

B. _____

C. _____

10. Basic life support (BLS) procedures support

_____.

11. _____ must

be started at once when a person is in cardiac arrest.

12. List the ABCs of CPR.

   A. _____

   B. _____

   C. _____

13. The airway is often obstructed during cardiac arrest.

   The _____

   opens the airway.

14. To check for adequate breathing, you must not take more than 10 seconds to:

   A. _____

   B. _____

   C. _____

   D. _____

   E. _____

15. When you start CPR, give _____

   first. During CPR, give _____ breaths

   after every _____ chest compressions.

16. Before starting chest compressions, check for a

   _____.

17. Explain how you would find the carotid pulse.

   _____

   _____

   _____

18. How far is the sternum depressed when doing chest compressions on an adult?

   _____

19. Chest compressions are given in a regular rhythm at a

   rate of _____.

20. Foreign-body airway obstruction (FBAO) can lead to

   _____.

21. List four factors that put older persons at risk for choking.

   A. _____

   B. _____

   C. _____

   D. _____

22. The _____ is

   used to relieve FBAO.

23. For which persons is the Heimlich maneuver not effective?

   _____

   _____

24. When is the recovery position used?

   _____

   _____

25. Do not use the recovery position if _____

   _____

   _____

   _____.

26. Describe ventricular fibrillation.

   _____

   _____

   _____

   _____

   _____

27. A _____ is used to deliver a shock

   to the heart. The shock stops the ventricular fibrilla-

   tion and allows the return of a regular heart rhythm.

28. With internal hemorrhage, bleeding occurs

_____

_____.

29. Bleeding from _____

occurs in spurts.

30. What should you do if direct pressure over the bleeding site does not control external bleeding?

_____

_____

_____

31. List seven signs and symptoms of shock.

A. _____

B. _____

C. _____

D. _____

E. _____

F. _____

G. _____

32. List seven causes of seizures.

A. _____

B. _____

C. _____

D. _____

E. _____

F. _____

G. _____

33. The two major types of seizures are

_____ and

_____.

34. Describe the two phases of a generalized tonic-clonic seizure (grand mal seizure).

A. _____

_____

_____

_____

B. _____

_____

_____

_____

35. Vomiting can be life-threatening because

_____

_____

_____

_____.

36. You need to observe vomitus for

_____

_____.

37. Vomitus that looks like coffee grounds, contains

_____.

38. Stroke occurs when _____

_____

_____.

39. Define these terms that can cause a stroke:

    A. Thrombus

    _____

    _____

    B. Embolus

    _____

    _____

    C. Hemorrhage

    _____

    _____

40. Signs of stroke depend on _____

    _____.

Circle the BEST Answer

41. When providing emergency care, it is important to do all of the following *except*
    A. Check for signs of life-threatening problems.
    B. Move the person to a comfortable position.
    C. Call for help.
    D. Keep the person warm.

42. The airway is opened by
    A. Turning the head to the side
    B. Lifting the head up and tilting forward
    C. Sitting the person up
    D. The head-tilt/chin-lift maneuver

43. During two-person cardiopulmonary resuscitation on an adult, which is correct?
    A. Give 1 breath after every 10 chest compressions.
    B. Give 2 breaths after every 15 chest compressions.
    C. Give 1 breath after every 5 chest compressions.
    D. Give 1 breath at the same rate as chest compressions.

44. For chest compressions to be effective, the person
    A. Must be in a sitting position
    B. Must be flat and on a soft surface
    C. Must be supine and on a hard, flat surface
    D. Is positioned with pillows

45. You determine unresponsiveness in an adult by
    A. Observing the person's color
    B. Feeling for a pulse
    C. Taking the person's blood pressure
    D. Tapping or gently shaking the person and asking, "Are you OK?"

46. If you find a person unconscious, you can assume that the cause is choking.
    A. True
    B. False

47. Internal hemorrhage is suspected. Which action is correct?
    A. Keep the person cool and in the semi-Fowler's position.
    B. Give the person cool water to drink.
    C. Apply pressure to the area.
    D. Call for help and keep the person warm.

48. Which is *not* a sign of shock?
    A. Rapid respirations
    B. High blood pressure
    C. Rapid and weak pulse
    D. Confusion

49. Which does *not* promote safety for a person during a generalized tonic-clonic seizure?
    A. Lower the person to the floor.
    B. Turn the person on his or her side.
    C. Restrain body movements during the seizure.
    D. Loosen tight clothing around the person's neck.

50. Emergency care for fainting includes all of the following *except*
    A. Loosen clothing
    B. Have the person sit or lie down.
    C. If the person is lying down, elevate the legs.
    D. Give the person something to eat.

Additional Learning Activities

1. Identify the agencies in your community that offer classes in basic life support procedures and first aid. The following list may be helpful:
   A. Hospitals
   B. Nursing centers
   C. Community colleges
   D. The American Heart Association
   E. The American Red Cross
   F. The National Safety Council

2. If possible, enroll in a basic life support class. Your instructor can help you with this process.

6 Promoting Residents' Rights and Independence

OBJECTIVES

The questions and student activities in this chapter will help you meet these objectives.

- Define the key terms listed in Chapter 6
- Identify the losses experienced by nursing center residents
- Describe residents' rights as required by OBRA
- Explain how you can promote the resident's rights
- Explain how to promote a resident's independence
- Identify the OBRA environment requirements that promote independence
- Explain how social activities promote independence
- Describe how the nursing team can promote a person's sexuality
- Explain the purpose of the Patient Self-Determination Act
- Describe the role of a long-term care ombudsman

Study Questions

Matching

Match each term with the correct definition.

1. _____ Someone who supports or promotes the needs and interests of another person

2. _____ The physical, psychological, social, cultural, and spiritual factors that affect a person's feelings and attitudes about sex

3. _____ A document stating a person's wishes about health care when that person cannot make his or her own decisions

4. _____ A document about measures that support or maintain life when death is likely

5. _____ Gives the power to make care decisions to another person

A. Living will

B. Advance directive

C. Durable power of attorney for health care

D. Sexuality

E. Ombudsman

Fill in the Blanks

6. Where do most older people live?

   _____

7. List five losses that may be experienced by a person entering a nursing center.

   A. _____

   B. _____

   C. _____

   D. _____

   E. _____

8. The health team helps persons cope with loss and improve their quality of life by _____

   _____

   _____.

9. Nursing centers must protect and promote

_____.

10. Ms. Genoa is a resident of Park View Nursing Center. She has dementia and is not able to exercise her rights. Who does so for her?

_____

_____

11. When are residents informed of their rights?

_____

_____

12. Mr. Majors is a resident at Park View Nursing Center. He tells you that he wants to see his medical record. What should you do?

_____

_____

13. Mr. Majors tells the nurse that he does not want oxygen therapy ordered by the doctor. Which right is Mr. Majors exercising?

_____

_____

14. Information about the person's care, treatment, and condition is kept _____.

15. Residents have the right to voice _____,

_____,

and _____ about treatment and care.

16. Involuntary seclusion is:

A. _____

B. _____

C. _____

17. Mr. Green's son has been visiting. Mr. Green has a bruise on his left cheek and is crying after his son leaves. What should you do?

_____

_____

18. Nursing centers cannot employ persons who were

convicted of _____

_____.

19. Some drugs are restraints because they affect

_____

_____.

20. Nursing centers must care for residents in a manner

that promotes _____

_____.

21. _____ and

_____ give persons

the right to accept or refuse treatment.

Circle the BEST Answer

22. The person has the right to be informed about his or her condition. The information must be given in the language the person understands.
A. True
B. False

23. The right to personal privacy involves all of the following *except*
A. Using the bathroom in private
B. Not exposing the person's body unnecessarily
C. Getting written permission from the resident before all care measures
D. Visiting with family and friends in private

24. The right to personal choice means
A. The person's doctor decides what is best for the person.
B. The doctor, nurse, and dietitian plan and decide the resident's care and treatment.
C. The person's bath schedule is set at the time of admission
D. Residents have the right to choose activities, schedules, and care based on their preferences.

25. Ms. Jones is a nursing center resident. She wants to help set the tables in the resident dining room for the noon meal. This is not allowed because residents cannot perform work in nursing centers.
    A. True
    B. False

26. Which is *not* a resident right? The right to
    A. Participate in resident and family groups
    B. Information about another resident's condition
    C. Keep and use personal items
    D. Voice disputes and grievances

27. You suspect that a resident has hidden bread and milk in his or her closet. You can search the closet without the person's permission.
    A. True
    B. False

28. Restraints require a doctor's order.
    A. True
    B. False

29. To promote resident independence
    A. Perform care measures as quickly as possible.
    B. Do as much as possible for the person.
    C. Keep the signal light within the person's reach.
    D. Provide all residents with special eating utensils.

30. Attitudes and sex needs stay the same throughout life.
    A. True
    B. False

31. A long-term care ombudsman
    A. Monitors nursing center care
    B. Is employed by the nursing center
    C. Writes nursing center policy
    D. Hires nursing center staff

32. Which action does *not* promote the residents' dignity?
    A. Using the right tone of voice
    B. Using good eye contact
    C. Calling the resident "Honey"
    D. Listening with interest to what the resident is saying

33. Which measure promotes privacy and self-determination?
    A. Using privacy curtains only when the resident requests it
    B. Keeping the door open during care measures
    C. Draping the person only if he or she has a roommate
    D. Knocking on the door before entering and waiting to be asked in

34. You may share resident information with any health team member.
    A. True
    B. False

35. Which is *not* an OBRA requirement?
    A. Recreational areas are comfortable for residents.
    B. Halls have handrails.
    C. Chairs vary in size to meet resident needs.
    D. Furniture is comfortable for staff.

36. Married couples living in nursing centers are allowed to share a room.
    A. True
    B. False

37. Which measure promotes the person's sexuality?
    A. Choosing the right clothing for the person
    B. Exposing the person during care
    C. Allowing privacy for masturbation
    D. Performing all grooming activities for the person

Additional Learning Activities

1. List some ways that you can help nursing center residents express their sexuality.

2. List some ways you express your sexuality.

3. Think about how it might feel if you were not allowed to do the things that help you express your sexuality.

4. Think about resident rights in relationship to your daily life.

   A. How important are these rights to you?

   B. How would you feel if your rights were limited or taken away?

5. Think about how you feel about advance directives. Write down your thoughts. Answer these questions:

   A. Do you know whom you would want to make decisions for you if you could not make your own decisions?

   B. How can you make sure your wishes are carried out?

7 Measurements

OBJECTIVES

The questions and student activities in this chapter will help you meet these objectives.
- Define the key terms listed in Chapter 7
- Explain why vital signs are measured
- List the factors affecting vital signs
- Identify the normal ranges for each temperature site
- Know when to use each temperature site
- Identify the pulse sites
- Describe normal respirations
- Describe the practices followed when measuring blood pressure
- Explain how to prepare the person for height and weight measurements
- Explain why intake and output are measured
- Identify the fluids counted as intake and the fluids counted as output
- Explain how to assist with pain assessment
- Perform the procedures described in Chapter 7

Study Questions

Matching

Match each term with the correct definition.

1. _____ The amount of force exerted against the walls of an artery by the blood

2. _____ The amount of heat in the body that is a balance between the amount of heat produced and the amount lost by the body

3. _____ A cuff and measuring device used to measure blood pressure

4. _____ The pressure in the arteries when the heart is at rest

5. _____ Systolic pressures that remain above 140 mm Hg and diastolic pressures that remain above 90 mm Hg

6. _____ The beat of the heart felt at an artery as a wave of blood passes through the artery

7. _____ When the systolic blood pressure is below 90 mm Hg and the diastolic pressure is below 60 mm Hg

8. _____ The number of heartbeats or pulses felt in 1 minute

9. _____ Breathing air into (inhalation) and out of (exhalation) the lungs

10. _____ The amount of force needed to pump blood out of the heart into the arterial circulation

11. _____ Temperature, pulse, respirations, and blood pressure

A. Sphygmomanometer

B. Hypertension

C. Blood pressure

D. Respiration

E. Pulse

F. Hypotension

G. Diastolic pressure

H. Pulse rate

I. Vital signs

J. Body temperature

K. Systolic pressure

Fill in the Blanks

12. Accuracy is essential when you _____,

    _____, and _____

    vital signs.

13. You are measuring Mr. Blue's vital signs. You are not sure of his blood pressure measurement. What should you do?

    _____

    _____

14. Vital signs show even minor changes in a person's condition. When measuring vital signs, you must report the following to the nurse at once:

    A. _____

    _____

    B. _____

    _____

    C. _____

    _____

15. List the sites for measuring body temperature.

    A. _____

    B. _____

    C. _____

    D. _____

16. Give the normal range of body temperatures in Fahrenheit and Centigrade for each of the following sites:

    A. Rectal

    _____

    _____

    B. Oral

    _____

    _____

17. Ms. Reed is unconscious and receiving oxygen. Which sites could be used to measure her temperature?

    _____

    _____

18. Rectal temperatures are not taken if the person has:

    A. _____

    B. _____

    C. _____

    D. _____

    E. _____

19. What information do you need from the nurse and the care plan before you take a person's temperature?

    A. _____

    B. _____

    C. _____

    D. _____

    E. _____

    F. _____

20. Why are rectal temperatures dangerous for persons with heart disease?

    _____

    _____

    _____

21. What should you do if a mercury glass thermometer breaks?

    _____

    _____

22. Which type of thermometer is lubricated before insertion?

    _____

23. You are taking an oral temperature. The person must

not _____,

_____,

_____, or

_____ for at least 15 to

20 minutes before you take his or her temperature.

24. For a rectal temperature, position the person in

_____ position.

25. Tympanic membrane thermometers measure tempera-

ture at the _____

_____.

26. Which site is most often used for taking a pulse?

_____

27. A _____ is an

instrument used to listen to sounds produced by the

heart, lungs, and other body organs.

28. Wipe the _____ and

_____ with anti-

septic wipes before and after using a stethoscope.

29. The rhythm of a pulse should be _____

_____.

30. Where is the radial pulse located?

_____

_____

31. Where is the apical pulse located?

_____

_____

32. You have taken a radial pulse on Mr. Lewis. What
observations do you need to report and record?

A. _____

B. _____

C. _____

33. Each respiration involves _____

_____

_____.

34. Normal respirations are _____,

_____, and regular.

Both sides of the chest _____

_____.

35. Why are respirations counted right after taking a pulse?

_____

_____

36. The period of heart muscle relaxation is called

_____.

37. A _____ and a _____

are used to measure blood pressure.

38. List the three types of sphygmomanometers.

A. _____

B. _____

C. _____

39. Do not take a blood pressure on an arm with:

A. _____

B. _____

C. _____

D. _____

E. _____

40. To deflate a blood pressure cuff, turn the valve

_____.

41. Why is it best to weigh a person before breakfast?

_____

_____

42. What information do you need from the nurse and the care plan before measuring height and weight?

A. _____

B. _____

43. Intake and output records are used to

_____

_____.

44. A measuring container for fluid is called

_____.

45. Why are Standard Precautions and the Bloodborne Pathogen Standard followed when measuring urine output?

_____

_____

46. Pain means to _____

_____.

47. Describe the following types of pain:

A. Acute pain

_____

_____

B. Phantom pain

_____

_____

48. Ms. Peters complains of pain in her right knee. What additional information about Ms. Peters' pain should you collect and report to the nurse?

A. _____

B. _____

C. _____

D. _____

E. _____

F. _____

49. List five body responses to pain.

A. _____

B. _____

C. _____

D. _____

E. _____

50. The circulatory system is made up of the

_____

_____.

51. Red blood cells are called _____

_____.

52. Platelets are needed for _____

_____.

53. The _____ is a

muscle that pumps blood through the blood vessels

to the tissues and cells.

54. How many chambers does the heart have?

_____

55. Which heart chamber receives blood from the lungs?

_____

56. _____ carry blood away from the heart.

57. The _____ is the largest artery.

58. _____ are the leading causes of death in the United States.

59. With _____ the resting blood pressure is too high.

60. Some drugs can lower blood pressure. List seven other measures that can help lower blood pressure.

   A. _____

   B. _____

   C. _____

   D. _____

   E. _____

   F. _____

   G. _____

61. Where are the coronary arteries located?

   _____

62. The major complications of CAD are:

   A. _____

   B. _____

63. _____ means chest pain.

64. Chest pain that is not relieved by rest and nitroglycerin may signal _____.

   The person needs _____

   _____.

65. With _____, part of the heart muscle dies from lack of blood flow to the heart muscle.

66. Heart failure or congestive heart failure occurs when _____

   _____.

67. With left-sided heart failure, blood backs up into the _____.

68. The _____ system brings oxygen into the lungs and removes carbon dioxide from them.

69. Oxygen and carbon dioxide are exchanged between the _____ and

   _____.

70. List the three disorders included under chronic obstructive pulmonary disease (COPD).

   A. _____

   B. _____

   C. _____

71. Pneumonia is _____

   _____

   _____.

72. List four causes of pneumonia.

   A. _____

   B. _____

   C. _____

   D. _____

73. Tuberculosis (TB) is spread by _____

   _____

   _____.

74. TB can be detected by _____

   _____.

Labeling

75. Label the pulse sites. Start with A at the top.

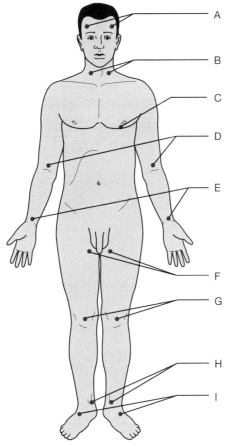

A. _____

B. _____

C. _____

D. _____

E. _____

F. _____

G. _____

H. _____

I. _____

76. Place an X at the apical pulse site.

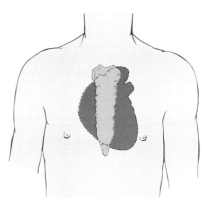

Circle the BEST Answer

77. Unless otherwise ordered, vital signs are taken
    A. After the person's bath
    B. With the person lying or sitting
    C. After breakfast
    D. After performing range-of-motion exercise

78. Do *not* take a tympanic membrane temperature if the person
    A. Is unconscious   C. Has ear drainage
    B. Has diarrhea   D. Has heart disease

79. You are taking a rectal temperature with a glass thermometer. Which is *incorrect?*
    A. Privacy is important.
    B. The thermometer is lubricated before insertion.
    C. The thermometer is held in place.
    D. The thermometer remains in the rectum for 1 minute.

80. Axillary temperatures
    A. Are more reliable than oral, rectal, or tympanic temperatures
    B. Are taken right after bathing the person
    C. Are taken for three minutes
    D. Are used when other routes cannot be used

81. Pulse rate is affected by
    A. Age   C. Pain
    B. Exercise   D. All of the above

82. The normal adult pulse rate is between
    A. 60 and 100 beats per minute
    B. 50 and 60 beats per minute
    C. 80 and 110 beats per minute
    D. 100 and 120 beats per minute

83. The force of a pulse relates to
    A. How regular the pulse is
    B. The strength of the pulse
    C. The number of beats per minute
    D. The number of skipped beats

84. Which adult blood pressure is reported to the nurse at once?
    A. 190/98   C. 120/80
    B. 130/82   D. 118/76

85. It is not necessary to report a blood pressure reading of 84/50 to the nurse because some people normally have low blood pressure.
    A. True
    B. False

86. You should ask the person to urinate after you weigh him or her.
    A. True
    B. False

87. Respiratory muscles weaken with aging.
    A. True
    B. False

Additional Learning Activities

1. Under the supervision of your instructor, practice the procedures in Chapter 7 with a classmate. Use the procedure checklists on pages 135-143 as a guide. Practice with various partners. Take your turn being the resident. Use a simulator for practicing rectal temperature.
   A. Temperature
      (1) Practice reading a glass thermometer.
      (2) If available, practice taking temperatures with different types of thermometers. List the advantages and disadvantages of each.
   B. Pulse
      (1) Practice with various classmates. Locate the following pulse sites: carotid, radial, brachial, popliteal, and dorsalis pedis.
      (2) Take radial pulses on various persons. Note the differences in rate, rhythm, and force.
      (3) Take a person's pulse before and after exercise. Notice and record the differences in rate, rhythm, and force.
   C. Respirations
      (1) Practice with various people. Note differences in respiratory rates. Note changes in the respiratory rate and depth of respirations with exercise.
   D. Blood pressure
      (1) Practice with various people.
      (2) Take and record blood pressure before and after exercise.
      (3) Take and record blood pressures with the person lying, sitting, and standing.
      (4) If available, practice using different types of blood pressure equipment. Discuss advantages and disadvantages of each.

2. Read the vignette. Answer the questions that follow.
   Mrs. Herman is a 75-year-old resident at Westlake Nursing Center. She has heart disease. She is also confused and restless. She has an intravenous (IV) infusion in her left arm. You have been assigned to measure Mrs. Herman's vital signs.

A. What temperature sites can you use? Explain.

B. Which arm will you use to take her blood pressure? Explain.

C. What information do you need from the nurse and the care plan before measuring:

   (1) Temperature

   (2) Pulse

   (3) Respirations

(4) Blood pressure

D. How will you protect Mrs. Herman's privacy when measuring her vital signs?

E. What observations do you need to report and record when measuring:

   (1) Temperature

   (2) Pulse

   (3) Respirations

   (4) Blood pressure

F. What are the normal ranges for Mrs. Herman's

   (1) Oral temperature

   (2) Pulse

   (3) Respirations

   (4) Blood pressure

3. Under the supervision of your instructor, practice the procedures for measuring height and weight and measuring intake and output. Use the checklists on pages 144-145 as a guide.

8 Care of the Resident's Environment

OBJECTIVES

The questions and student activities in this chapter will help you meet these objectives.
- Define the key terms listed in Chapter 8
- Explain how to keep the resident's unit clean and safe
- Describe how to control temperature, odors, noise, and lighting
- Describe how to use furniture and equipment in the person's unit
- Describe open, closed, occupied, and surgical beds
- Explain the purpose of plastic and cotton drawsheets
- Handle linens following the rules of medical asepsis
- Perform the procedures described in Chapter 8

Study Questions

Matching

Match each term with the correct definition.

1. _____ Having the means to be completely free from public view while in bed

2. _____ The head of the bed is raised, and the foot of the bed is lowered

3. _____ The head of the bed is raised 30 degrees, or the head of the bed is raised 30 degrees and the knee portion is raised 15 degrees

4. _____ The head of the bed is lowered, and the foot of the bed is raised

5. _____ A semi-sitting position; the head of the bed is raised 45 to 90 degrees

A. Reverse-Trendelenburg's position

B. Full visual privacy

C. Semi-Fowler's position

D. Fowler's position

E. Trendelenburg's position

Fill in the Blanks

6. Resident rooms are designed for

_____,

_____,

and _____.

7. The resident unit is considered

_____. It is treated like

_____.

8. What is the temperature range required by the Omnibus Budget Reconciliation Act of 1987 (OBRA)?

_____

9. Drafts occur as air moves. To protect persons from drafts, you need to

A. _____

B. _____

C. _____

D. _____

10. List four ways to control odors.

    A. _____

    B. _____

    C. _____

    D. _____

11. Staff can reduce noise and increase resident comfort by:

    A. _____

    B. _____

    C. _____

    D. _____

12. Good lighting is needed for _____

    and _____.

13. Keeping light controls within the person's reach pro-

    tects the person's right to _____

    _____.

14. Why are hospital beds raised to give care?

    _____

    _____

15. Manual beds have cranks at the foot of the bed. Why are these cranks kept down when not in use?

    _____

    _____

16. Which bed positions require a doctor's order?

    A. _____

    B. _____

17. When must bed wheels be locked?

    _____

    _____

18. Never place _____,

    _____, or

    _____ on the overbed table.

19. What is the purpose of the privacy curtain?

    _____

    _____

    _____

20. What is the purpose of the grab bars by the toilet in a resident's bathroom?

    _____

    _____

    _____

21. OBRA requires that each resident have closet space

    with _____

    and _____.

22. Describe four ways to make a bed.

    A. _____

    _____

    B. _____

    _____

    C. _____

    _____

    D. _____

    _____

23. Place clean linens on a _____

    _____.

24. When removing dirty linens from the bed,

    _____.

    Roll each piece _____.

25. When are wet, damp, or soiled linens changed?

    _____

26. What is the purpose of a cotton drawsheet?

    _____

    _____

27. What information do you need from the nurse and the care plan before making a bed?

    A. _____

    B. _____

    C. _____

    D. _____

    E. _____

28. Why is it important to wear gloves when removing linen from the person's bed?

    _____

    _____

29. After making a bed, you must _____

    _____

    _____.

30. You are putting the top sheet on a closed bed. The

    hem stitching should face _____

    _____.

31. Describe how you should place the pillow on the person's bed.

    _____

    _____

32. How often do you need to straighten a person's bed linens?

    _____

Circle the BEST Answer

33. Which room temperature range is usually comfortable for most healthy people?
    A. 68° F to 74° F
    B. 71° F to 81° F
    C. 65° F to 68° F
    D. 82° F to 90° F

34. You are making a closed bed for a new resident. Which piece of linen is placed on the bed first?
    A. Bottom sheet
    B. Cotton draw sheet
    C. Mattress pad
    D. Pillow case

35. What type of bed is made after a person is discharged?
    A. An open bed
    B. A closed bed
    C. An occupied bed
    D. A surgical bed

36. You are making an occupied bed. Which is *incorrect?*
    A. Keep the bed in the lowest position.
    B. If the person uses bed rails, the far bed rail is up.
    C. Keep the person in good alignment.
    D. After making the bed, lock the bed wheels.

37. You have finished making a surgical bed for a resident arriving by stretcher. You should leave the bed in its highest position.
    A. True
    B. False

38. Which is a rule for bed making?
    A. Follow the rules for sterile technique.
    B. Shake linens to remove wrinkles.
    C. Hold linens against your uniform.
    D. Use good body mechanics at all times.

39. You brought an extra pillowcase into a resident room. What should you do?
    A. Take it back to the linen closet.
    B. Put it in the dirty laundry.
    C. Use it for another resident.
    D. Put it in the resident's closet.

40. Lighting, temperature, and ventilation are adjusted for staff comfort.
    A. True
    B. False

41. The overbed table is used for meals, writing, reading, and other activities.
    A. True
    B. False

42. OBRA requires a unit to have at least one comfortable chair for personal and visitor use.
   A. True
   B. False

43. You may search a person's closet and drawers without the person's permission.
   A. True
   B. False

Additional Learning Activities

1. How important is your personal space to you?

   A. How would you feel about sharing one room with another person?

   B. How would you decide which items to take with you and which items to leave behind?

2. Practice gathering linen in the correct order for bed-making. List the correct order on an index card. Carry the card with you until you have the order memorized.

3. Practice the procedures in Chapter 8. Use the procedure checklists provided on pages 146-151.

4. Observe classmates performing the procedures in Chapter 8. Use the procedure checklists provided on pages 146-151.

9 Observing, Reporting, and Recording

OBJECTIVES

The questions and student activities in this chapter will help you meet these objectives.
- Define the key terms listed in Chapter 9
- Explain the difference between objective and subjective data
- Identify the observations that you need to report to the nurse
- List the basic rules for recording
- Explain the purpose, parts, and information found in the medical record
- Describe the legal and ethical aspects of medical records
- Explain how computers are used in health care
- Explain how to protect the right to privacy when using computers
- Use the 24-hour clock, medical terminology, and abbreviations

Study Questions

Matching

Match each term with the correct definition.

1. _____ Objective data

2. _____ The oral account of care and observations

3. _____ A written account of a person's condition and response to treatment and care

4. _____ A word element placed before a root. It changes the meaning of the word.

5. _____ A word element containing the basic meaning of the word

6. _____ A word element placed after a root. It changes the meaning of the word.

7. _____ Using the senses of sight, hearing, touch, and smell to collect information

8. _____ Things a person tells you about that you cannot observe through your senses (symptoms)

9. _____ Information that is seen, heard, felt, or smelled

10. _____ The written account of care and observations (charting)

A. Observation

B. Prefix

C. Medical record

D. Objective data

E. Suffix

F. Recording

G. Root

H. Signs

I. Reporting

J. Subjective data

Fill in the Blanks

11. You have made an error when charting on the medical record. What should you do?

_____

_____

_____

12. When should you chart a procedure or treatment?

_____

_____

13. Why is it important to chart safety measures such as placing the signal light within reach?

_____

_____

14. The nursing center you work in uses computers. Why is it important not to give anyone your password?

_____

_____

_____

_____

15. The health team communicates by _____

_____.

16. When should you report changes in the person's condition?

_____

17. What is the purpose of end-of-shift report?

_____

_____

_____

18. The medical record is a _____,

_____ document.

19. If you have access to the medical record, you must

keep information _____.

20. If you are not involved in the person's care, you have

no right to review the chart. To do so is

_____.

21. Anyone who reads your charting should know:

A. _____

B. _____

C. _____

22. Enter "**o**" for objective data and "**s**" for subjective data.
    A. _____ Pain
    B. _____ Nausea
    C. _____ Vomiting
    D. _____ Dizziness
    E. _____ Clear yellow urine
    F. _____ Warm moist skin
    G. _____ Numbness
    H. _____ Pulse rate of 80 beats per minute

23. Convert the following times from standard time to 24-hour clock time.

    A. 6:15 PM _____

    B. 8:00 AM _____

    C. 2:30 PM _____

    D. 5:02 PM _____

    E. 10:55 AM _____

    F. 1:29 PM _____

    G. 1:33 AM _____

    H. 9:00 PM _____

24. Convert the following times from 24-hour clock time to standard time.

    A. 1600 _____

    B. 0945 _____

    C. 1115 _____

    D. 2120 _____

    E. 1705 _____

25. _____ are used

    to record frequent measurements or observations.

26. Which form would you use to record a resident's complaint of nausea?

    _____

27. Define the following directional terms:

    A. Anterior (ventral)

       _____

       _____

    B. Lateral

       _____

       _____

    C. Posterior (dorsal)

       _____

       _____

    D. Proximal

       _____

       _____

28. Abbreviations are _____

    _____.

29. What should you do if you are unsure of an abbreviation?

    _____

    _____

30. What do the following abbreviations mean?

    A. NPO _____

    B. VS _____

    C. ml _____

    D. STAT _____

Circle the BEST Answer

31. Who has access to a person's medical record?
    A. The person's family members
    B. Health team members involved in the person's care
    C. Laundry personnel
    D. Visitors

32. You are reporting resident care. Which is *incorrect?*
    A. Report your observations to the nurse.
    B. Report the care that was given by a co-worker.
    C. Reports must be prompt, thorough, and accurate.
    D. Report any changes from normal at once.

33. When recording, you should do all of the following *except*
    A. Use ink.
    B. Make sure writing is legible and neat.
    C. Use correct spelling and grammar.
    D. Use correcting fluid if you make a mistake.

34. The intake and output (I&O) record is one type of
    A. Flow sheet
    B. Subjective data
    C. Admission sheet
    D. Progress note

35. Computers are often used in health care. Which is *false?*
    A. Computers save time.
    B. The right to privacy must be protected.
    C. The center has the right to monitor your computer use.
    D. E-mail is used for information that requires immediate reporting.

36. What does the medical term *gastritis* mean?
    A. Difficulty urinating
    B. Nerve pain
    C. Inflammation of the stomach
    D. Excision of the ovary

37. Which medical term means study of the skin?
    A. Bronchitis
    B. Dermatology
    C. Neuralgia
    D. Encephalopathy

38. Myalgia means
    A. Nausea
    B. Heart disease
    C. Muscle pain
    D. Eye drainage

Additional Learning Activities

1. Practice your observation, recording, and reporting skills. Ask a classmate or member of your family to help.
   A. Talk to the person for about 5 minutes. Then record the following information:

      (1) Color and length of hair

      (2) Color of eyes

      (3) Description of any jewelry the person is wearing

      (4) Description of clothing the person is wearing

      (5) Any special features (birthmarks, scars, etc.)

      (6) Any information the person gave you about him or herself

   B. Use a note pad to record your observations.

   C. Use your notes to give a verbal report.

   D. Discuss the accuracy of what you recorded and reported about the person and the conversation.

2. Make flash cards of the prefixes, root words, and suffixes in Chapter 9. Write the meaning of each on the back of each flash card. Use the flash cards to help you study and learn medical terms. You can work alone or with a classmate.

3. Make flash cards of the common abbreviations located on the inside of the back cover in the textbook. Use these to help you study and memorize common abbreviations.

10 The Dying Person

OBJECTIVES

The questions and student activities in this chapter will help you meet these objectives.
- Define the key terms listed in Chapter 10
- Explain how religion, culture, and age affect attitudes about death
- Describe the five stages of dying
- Explain how to meet the needs of the dying person and family
- Explain how people can legally express their end-of-life wishes
- Identify the signs of approaching death and the signs of death
- Perform the procedure described in Chapter 10

Study Questions

Matching

Match each term with the correct definition.

1. _____ After death

2. _____ A tumor that grows slowly and within a local area

3. _____ The stiffness or rigidity of skeletal muscles that occurs after death

4. _____ The spread of cancer to other body parts

5. _____ An order written by the doctor after consulting with the person and the family. It means the person will not be resuscitated.

6. _____ An illness or injury for which there is no reasonable expectation of recovery

A. "Do Not Resuscitate" order

B. Postmortem

C. Rigor mortis

D. Benign tumor

E. Terminal illness

F. Metastasis

Fill in the Blanks

7. Hospice care focuses on _____

_____

_____.

8. The goal of hospice care is to _____

_____

_____.

9. _____ is the

belief that the spirit or soul is reborn in another body

or in another form of life.

10. List five things adults may fear when facing death.

    A. _____

    B. _____

    C. _____

    D. _____

    E. _____

11. List the five stages of dying described by Dr. Elisabeth Kübler-Ross.

    A. _____

    B. _____

    C. _____

    D. _____

    E. _____

12. Why are listening and touch important care measures for the dying person?

    _____

    _____

    _____

    _____

    _____

13. As death nears, _____ is one of the last functions to be lost.

14. The dying person's room should be _____

    _____

    _____.

15. The dying person's family needs _____

    _____

    _____.

16. List six signs that death is near.

    A. _____

    B. _____

    C. _____

    D. _____

    E. _____

    F. _____

17. The signs of death include:

    A. _____

    B. _____

18. Which health team member pronounces the person dead?

    _____

19. When does postmortem care begin?

    _____

    _____

20. _____ and

    _____ are

    followed when giving postmortem care.

Circle the BEST Answer

21. Attitudes and beliefs about death usually stay the same throughout a person's life.
    A. True
    B. False

22. Seven-year-olds know death is final.
    A. True
    B. False

23. Children between the ages of three and five
    A. Know that death is final
    B. Often think they will die
    C. Think death is punishment for being bad
    D. Are not curious about death

24. The person in the bargaining stage of dying
    A. Is very sad
    B. Makes promises in exchange for more time
    C. Is calm and at peace
    D. Feels anger and rage

25. A new growth of abnormal cells is called
    A. Benign
    B. A lump
    C. A tumor
    D. Cancer

26. Which is *not* a cancer risk factor?
    A. A high-fiber diet
    B. Smoking tobacco
    C. Close relatives with certain types of cancer
    D. Exposure to radiation

27. Radiation therapy kills cancer cells and normal cells.
    A. True
    B. False

28. Stomatitis is
    A. Chemotherapy
    B. Loss of appetite
    C. A malignant tumor
    D. Inflammation of the mouth

29. Surgery is done to
    A. Cure or control cancer
    B. Remove tumors
    C. Relieve pain from advanced cancer
    D. All of the above are correct.

30. Ms. Roberts is dying. She asks you to stay and talk in the middle of the night. Which is *correct?*
    A. Tell her that she needs to sleep.
    B. Call her family to stay with her.
    C. Call a pastor to talk with her.
    D. Being there and listening help to meet her psychological and social needs.

31. You promote comfort when caring for a dying person by
    A. Keeping the room dark
    B. Whispering when in the person's presence
    C. Providing good skin care and personal hygiene
    D. Avoiding touch

32. You help the family of the dying person by doing all of the following *except*
    A. Being available, considerate, and courteous
    B. Using touch to show your concern
    C. Enforcing visiting hours
    D. Respecting the right to privacy

33. Postmortem care involves all of the following *except*
    A. Pronouncing the person dead
    B. Positioning the body in normal alignment before rigor mortis sets in
    C. Preparing the body for viewing by the family
    D. Bathing soiled areas

34. It is not necessary to provide privacy when doing postmortem care because the person is dead.
    A. True
    B. False

Additional Learning Activities

1. List your thoughts and feelings about death and dying. Answer these questions:
   A. How do your religion, culture, and age affect your feelings about death?
   B. Have you had experience with the death of a family member or friend that affects your feelings about death and dying? Explain.

2. List ways you can help the family and friends of a dying person.
   A. What needs might they have?
   B. What fears might they have?

C. What support systems are available?

3. Do you have fears about caring for dying persons? Discuss them with your instructor.

   A. How might you deal with your feelings and fears?

D. What are the roles of various members of the health care team in providing support and comfort?

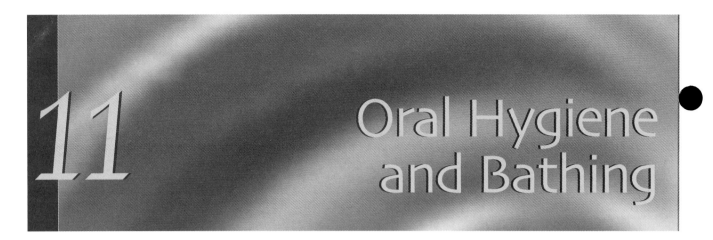

11

Oral Hygiene and Bathing

OBJECTIVES

The questions and student activities in this chapter will help you meet these objectives.
- Define the key terms listed in Chapter 11
- Describe the care given before and after breakfast, after lunch, and in the evening

- Explain the importance of oral hygiene and bathing
- Identify the safety measures for tub baths and showers
- Explain the purposes of a back massage
- Explain the purposes of perineal care
- Perform the procedures described in Chapter 11

Study Questions

Matching

Match each term with the correct definition.

1. _____ Care given before breakfast

2. _____ Involves washing the person's body in bed

3. _____ Care given before bedtime

4. _____ Mouth care

5. _____ Cleaning the genital and anal areas

6. _____ Care given after breakfast

7. _____ Involves bathing the person's face, hands, axillae, back, buttocks, and perineal area

A. Complete bed bath

B. Morning care

C. Perineal care

D. Partial bath

E. Early morning care (AM care)

F. Evening care (PM care)

G. Oral hygiene

Fill in the Blanks

8. Intact skin prevents _____ from entering the body.

9. Which culture does not allow cold water to be added to hot water?

_____

10. Oral hygiene does the following:

A. _____

B. _____

C. _____

D. _____

E. _____

11. What type of toothbrush is used to brush a person's teeth?

    _____

12. What information do you need from the nurse and the care plan before you assist with oral hygiene?

    A. _____

    B. _____

    C. _____

    D. _____

    E. _____

    F. _____

13. List three reasons to follow Standard Precautions and the Bloodborne Pathogen Standard when giving oral hygiene.

    A. _____

    B. _____

    C. _____

14. Oral hygiene is given at the following times:

    A. _____

    B. _____

    C. _____

15. Dry mouth is common from

    _____,

    _____,

    _____, and

    _____.

16. You are giving oral care to an unconscious person. You need to protect the person from aspiration. How should you position the person?

    _____

    _____

17. During cleaning, firmly hold dentures

    _____

    _____

    _____.

18. You have finished cleaning Ms. Barnett's dentures. She will not wear them until morning. How will you store them?

    _____

    _____

19. Complete or partial bed baths, tub baths, or showers are given. The method used depends on:

    A. _____

    B. _____

    C. _____

20. List six reasons that bathing is important.

    A. _____

    B. _____

    C. _____

    D. _____

    E. _____

    F. _____

21. Water temperature for a complete bed bath is usually

    _____

    _____ for adults.

22. You have finished giving Mr. Vance a bath. What observations do you need to report and record?

   A. _____

   B. _____

   C. _____

   D. _____

   E. _____

   F. _____

   G. _____

   H. _____

   I. _____

   J. _____

23. Why is powder not used near persons with respiratory disorders?

   _____

   _____

24. List three risks from tub baths.

   A. _____

   B. _____

   C. _____

25. You observe the skin when giving a back massage. What observations do you need to report and record?

   A. _____

   B. _____

   C. _____

26. When giving a back massage, you do not massage

   bony areas that are reddened because

   _____

   _____

   _____ .

27. Perineal care involves cleaning the genital and anal areas. Why is this important?

   _____

   _____

28. When is perineal care given?

   A. _____

   B. _____

29. When giving perineal care, you work from the

   cleanest area to the dirtiest. This means that you clean

   from the _____

   to the _____ .

30. You have finished giving perineal care to Ms. Ruiz. What observations do you need to report and record?

   A. _____

   B. _____

   C. _____

   D. _____

31. When giving perineal care, to protect yourself and

   the person from infection, you need to follow

   _____ and _____ .

Circle the BEST Answer

32. After giving oral hygiene, you need to report all of the following to the nurse *except*
   A. The type of toothbrush you used
   B. Dry, cracked, swollen, or blistered lips
   C. Mouth or breath odor
   D. Loose teeth

33. Use a toothbrush with soft bristles to brush the person's teeth.
   A. True
   B. False

34. When providing mouth care to the unconscious person, you need to
    A. Use your fingers to hold the mouth open.
    B. Position the person on his or her back.
    C. Explain what you are doing step by step.
    D. Avoid talking to the person.

35. How often is mouth care given to the unconscious person?
    A. At least every two hours
    B. Twice a day
    C. Every four hours
    D. Every six hours

36. When cleaning dentures, you need to
    A. Use hot water.
    B. Wear gloves.
    C. Store them dry in a container with a lid.
    D. Wrap them in a paper towel and place them in the bedside stand.

37. Which statement about bathing an older person is *true?*
    A. A complete bath is needed daily.
    B. Always use soap.
    C. Thorough rinsing is needed when using soap.
    D. Bath oils are used for tub baths.

38. To apply powder safely, do the following *except*
    A. Avoid shaking or sprinkling powder onto the person.
    B. Turn away from the person.
    C. Sprinkle a small amount of powder onto your hand or a cloth.
    D. Apply the powder in a thick layer.

39. You give Mr. Jones a complete bed bath. Do all of the following *except*
    A. Expose only the body part needed.
    B. Change the water if it is soapy or cool.
    C. Provide for privacy.
    D. Place the bed in the lowest horizontal position.

40. You are giving Ms. Gomez a tub bath. Which is *true?*
    A. The bath may cause Ms. Gomez to feel faint, weak, or tired.
    B. Turn hot water on first, then cold water.
    C. The bath should last 30 minutes.
    D. Fill the tub after Ms. Gomez gets into the tub.

41. After a tub bath, the person's skin is rubbed dry with a soft bath towel.
    A. True
    B. False

42. Which is *not* a safety measure for tub baths and showers?
    A. Clean the tub before and after use.
    B. Place a bath mat in the tub or on the shower floor if they do not have nonskid surfaces.
    C. Have the person use towel bars for support when getting in and out of the tub.
    D. Direct water away from the person while adjusting water temperature and pressure.

43. You need to drain the tub before the person gets out of the tub.
    A. True
    B. False

44. When giving a back massage, you need to do all of the following *except*
    A. Position the person in Fowler's position.
    B. Warm the lotion before applying it.
    C. Use firm strokes.
    D. Always keep your hands in contact with the person's skin.

45. A back massage is safe for all persons.
    A. True
    B. False

Additional Learning Activities

1. Discuss the importance of hygiene and cleanliness in your personal life. Answer these questions.
   A. How important is it for you to feel clean and free from unpleasant odors when you are around other people? Explain.
   B. What care routines do you practice daily to promote your cleanliness?

2. Have injuries or illnesses ever prevented you from carrying out your daily hygiene routines? Explain.

   A. Discuss how this affected your personal comfort.

   B. Discuss how your experiences might help you meet the hygiene needs of the persons you care for.

3. The procedures in this chapter require you to provide personal care to another person. They must be performed in a way that respects the person's privacy and dignity. It will help you to understand how the person feels if you practice the procedures with a classmate. Take your turn being the resident. Under the supervision of your instructor, use the procedure checklists provided on pages 154-169 to practice the procedures in Chapter 11. Use a simulator to practice female and male perineal care.

   A. After practicing each procedure, discuss your experience.

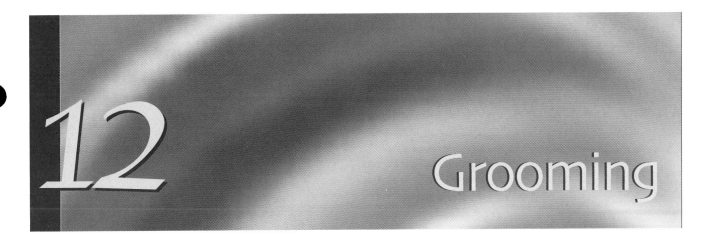

12 Grooming

OBJECTIVES

The questions and student activities in this chapter will help you meet these objectives.
- Define the key terms listed in Chapter 12
- Explain the importance of hair care, shaving, and nail and foot care

- Describe the safety measures for shaving a person
- Describe the rules for changing gowns and clothing
- Perform the procedures described in Chapter 12

Study Questions

Matching

Match each term with the correct definition.

1. _____ Hair loss

2. _____ The excessive amount of dry, white flakes from the scalp

3. _____ The infestation with lice

4. _____ The infestation of the scalp with lice

5. _____ The infestation of the body with lice

6. _____ Excessive body hair in women and children

7. _____ The infestation of the pubic hair with lice

A. Pediculosis corporis

B. Hirsutism

C. Alopecia

D. Pediculosis capitis

E. Pediculosis pubis

F. Pediculosis

G. Dandruff

Fill in the Blanks

8. You assist with daily hair care. The care plan reflects

   the person's _____,

   _____,

   _____,

   _____,

   and _____.

9. Male pattern baldness occurs with aging and is due to

   _____.

10. Ms. Granger is a nursing center resident. Who chooses how to brush, comb, and style her hair?

   _____

11. When brushing and combing hair, start at the

    _____. Then brush or

    comb to the _____.

12. To brush or comb through matted or tangled hair you need to:

    A. _____

    B. _____

    C. _____

    D. _____

    E. _____

13. How would you comb curly hair?

    _____

    _____

    _____

    _____

    _____

    _____

14. You are assisting Mr. Crane with hair care. What observations do you need to report and record?

    A. _____

    B. _____

    C. _____

    D. _____

    E. _____

15. List four shampooing methods.

    A. _____

    B. _____

    C. _____

    D. _____

16. The shampoo method depends on:

    A. _____

    B. _____

    C. _____

17. What information do you need from the nurse and the care plan before shampooing hair?

    A. _____

    B. _____

    C. _____

    D. _____

    E. _____

    F. _____

    G. _____

18. You used a medicated shampoo for Ms. Martin. What should you do with the shampoo when you are finished shampooing Ms. Martin's hair?

    _____

19. Mr. James is 80 years old. He cannot tip his head back. You are shampooing his hair in the tub. How would you keep soap out of his eyes while shampooing his hair?

    _____

    _____

    _____

    _____

    _____

20. Water temperature for shampooing should be about

    _____.

21. Safety razors (blade razors) are not used for the following persons:

    A. _____

    B. _____

22. Where are used razor blades and disposable shavers discarded?

_____

23. Nail and foot care prevents _____,

_____, and _____.

24. You are giving nail and foot care to Mr. Lopez. What observations do you need to report and record?

A. _____

B. _____

C. _____

D. _____

E. _____

25. You are changing Mr. Parson's shirt. He has a paralyzed right arm. From which side should you remove his shirt first?

_____

26. What information do you need from the nurse and the care plan before changing clothing?

A. _____

B. _____

C. _____

D. _____

27. You are changing Ms. Green's standard gown. She has an IV in her right arm. She has an IV pump. What safety precaution do you need to follow?

_____

_____

Circle the BEST Answer

28. Brushing and combing hair is
    A. Part of early morning care, morning care, and afternoon care
    B. Done when you have time
    C. Not your responsibility
    D. Always done by the resident

29. When giving hair care, you need to
    A. Decide how to style the hair.
    B. Cut matted and tangled hair.
    C. Braid long hair to keep it neat.
    D. Start at the scalp and brush toward the hair ends.

30. A person receives a cut during shaving, you need to
    A. Report to the nurse only if you cannot stop the bleeding
    B. Apply direct pressure to the cut
    C. Put a bandage on the cut
    D. Apply an antibiotic ointment to the cut

31. Which is *not* a rule for shaving?
    A. Soften the skin before shaving.
    B. Hold the skin taut as necessary.
    C. Shave against the direction of hair growth when shaving the face and underarms.
    D. Rinse the body part thoroughly.

32. Mr. White has a beard. You do all of the following *except*
    A. Trim the beard once a week.
    B. Wash and comb the beard daily.
    C. Ask Mr. White how to groom his beard.
    D. Wash the beard whenever mouth or nose drainage is present.

33. When trimming fingernails, you
    A. Let the fingernails soak for 30 minutes before starting.
    B. Clip the fingernails in a curved shape.
    C. Be careful not to damage surrounding tissue.
    D. Use a scissors.

34. You do not cut or trim toenails if a person has diabetes.
    A. True
    B. False

35. You are giving foot care to Mr. Lopez. You must *not* apply lotion between his toes.
    A. True
    B. False

36. Which statement about changing clothing and gowns is *false?*
    A. Provide for privacy. Do not expose the person.
    B. Encourage the person to do as much as possible.
    C. Let the person choose what to wear.
    D. Put clothing on the strong side first.

37. Mr. Brown has an IV in his left arm. You need to
    A. Remove the gown from his right arm first.
    B. Remove the gown from his left arm first.
    C. Ask him which arm to remove first.
    D. Remove the gown from the side easiest for you to reach.

Additional Learning Activities

1. List the grooming activities you perform every day. Answer these questions.
    A. How important are your grooming routines?

    B. How important is personal choice when you are performing your grooming activities?

    C. How important is privacy when you are performing your grooming activities?

    D. How would you feel if you were unable to perform your grooming activities?
        (1) How would you want to be treated?

2. Read the vignette; then answer the questions that follow.
    Mr. Benson is a nursing center resident. He has weakness on his left side. He is taking a drug that slows blood clotting. You will be shaving him. You will also remove his gown and dress him for the day. He is able to follow directions and assist with his care.

    A. What type of razor will you use? Explain.

    B. What items do you need to collect to shave Mr. Benson?

    C. What safety measures will you practice when shaving Mr. Benson?

    D. How will you provide for Mr. Benson's privacy?

    E. What will you do when you finish the procedure?

    F. What information do you need from the nurse and the care plan before you dress Mr. Benson?

G. How will you remove Mr. Benson's gown?

A. What additional information do you need from the nurse and the care plan before you shampoo Ms. Dunn's hair?

H. How will you promote Mr. Benson's right to personal choice?

B. Can you use the shampoo that Ms. Dunn brought from home? Explain.

I. Mr. Benson has chosen a shirt that buttons in the front. How will you put on the shirt?

C. How can you promote Ms. Dunn's right to personal choice?

J. How will you put on Mr. Benson's pants?

D. What safety measures will you practice when shampooing Ms. Dunn's hair?

K. What will you do when you finish the procedure?

E. How will you keep shampoo out of Ms. Dunn's eyes?

3. Read the vignette; then answer the questions that follow.
   Ms. Dunn is an 80-year-old nursing center resident. You will be shampooing her hair during her tub bath. She wants to use the shampoo she brought from home. The nurse tells you that Ms. Dunn has an open area the size of a dime on top of her head.
   Ms. Dunn has arthritis and is unable to tip her head back.

F. How will you promote Ms. Dunn's right to privacy?

G. What observations do you need to report and record?

4. Carefully review the procedures in Chapter 12. Under the supervision of your instructor, use the procedure checklists on pages 173-187 to practice each procedure.
   A. Practice dressing and undressing procedures with classmates or family members.

   (1) Use different types of clothing (for example, clothes that open in front and clothes that open in back, button and pullover shirts, pants with zippers and buttons, and pants that pull on).

   (2) Role-play weakness on one side of the body.

   (3) Role-play that the person is not able to help.

   (4) Take your turn being the resident.

B. Discuss the experience.

   (1) How will your experience affect how you help others with grooming and dressing activities?

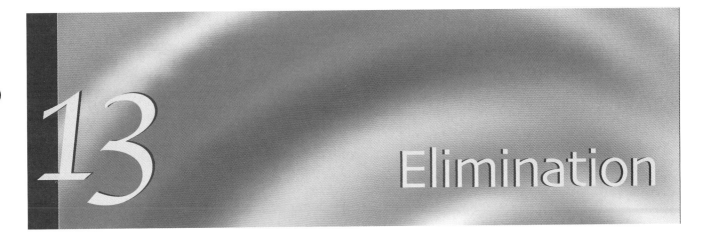

13 Elimination

OBJECTIVES

The questions and student activities in this chapter will help you meet these objectives.
- Define the key terms listed in Chapter 13
- Describe the structures and functions of the urinary and gastrointestinal systems
- Explain how aging affects the urinary and gastrointestinal systems
- Describe the common disorders of the urinary and gastrointestinal systems
- Describe measures that promote elimination
- List the observations to make about urine and bowel movements
- Describe urinary incontinence and the care required
- Explain how to care for persons with catheters
- Describe the methods for bladder and bowel training
- Explain how to collect urine and stool specimens
- Describe the purpose, solutions, and methods of enema administration
- Describe how to care for a person with an ostomy
- Perform the procedures described in Chapter 13

Study Questions

Crossword

Across
4. Scant amount of urine
7. Blood in the urine
8. The process of emptying urine from the bladder

Down
1. Frequent urination at night
2. Urination
3. Abnormally large amounts of urine
5. Painful or difficult urination
6. A tube used to drain or inject fluid through a body opening

Crossword

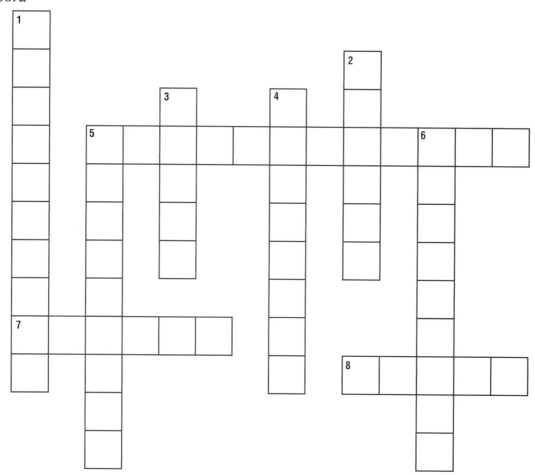

Across
5. The passage of a hard, dry stool
7. A surgically created opening
8. An opening

Down
1. The process of excreting feces from the rectum through the anus
2. Gas or air passed through the anus
3. The introduction of fluid into the rectum and lower colon
4. The frequent passage of liquid stools
5. A surgically created opening between the colon and the abdominal wall
6. A surgically created opening between the ileum and the abdominal wall

Matching

Match each term with the correct definition.

1. _____ Urine leaks during exercise and certain movements.

2. _____ Urine leaks when the bladder is too full.

3. _____ The person has bladder control but cannot use the toilet in time.

4. _____ The prolonged retention and buildup of feces in the rectum

5. _____ The excessive formation of gas in the stomach and intestines

6. _____ Loss of urine at predictable intervals; urine is lost when the bladder is full.

7. _____ Voiding at frequent intervals

8. _____ The loss of bladder control

9. _____ Excreted feces

10. _____ There is loss of urine in response to a sudden, urgent need to void.

11. _____ The inability to control the passage of feces and gas through the anus

12. _____ The need to void at once

13. _____ The semisolid mass of waste products in the colon that are expelled through the anus

A. Overflow incontinence

B. Flatulence

C. Urinary frequency

D. Functional incontinence

E. Urinary urgency

F. Stool

G. Fecal incontinence

H. Stress incontinence

I. Feces

J. Reflex incontinence

K. Urge incontinence

L. Urinary incontinence

M. Fecal impaction

Fill in the Blanks

14. The urinary system removes

_____

from the blood and maintains the body's

_____ .

15. The _____

removes solid wastes from the body.

16. List seven factors affecting urine production.

A. _____

B. _____

C. _____

D. _____

E. _____

F. _____

G. _____

17. _____ is when

the person does not empty the bladder completely.

Urine is left in the bladder after voiding.

18. List five common causes of urinary tract infections (UTIs).

    A. _____

    B. _____

    C. _____

    D. _____

    E. _____

19. Why are women at high risk for UTIs?

    _____

    _____

20. _____,

    _____,

    and _____ are

    risk factors for renal calculi.

21. List six signs and symptoms of cystitis.

    A. _____

    B. _____

    C. _____

    D. _____

    E. _____

    F. _____

22. With _____ the

    kidneys do not function or are severely impaired.

    Waste products are not removed from the blood.

23. You need to observe urine for

    _____,

    _____,

    _____,

    _____,

    and _____.

24. Mr. Lane has had hip replacement surgery. What type of bedpan should he use?

    _____

25. What information do you need from the nurse before assisting with the bedpan?

    A. _____

    B. _____

    C. _____

    D. _____

26. Follow _____

    and _____

    when handling bedpans, urinals, and their contents.

27. Men use _____ to void.

28. Why do you need to empty urinals promptly?

    A. _____

    B. _____

    C. _____

29. A _____ is a chair or

    wheelchair with an opening for a bedpan or container.

30. Ms. Harold has stress incontinence and urge incontinence. This is called _____

    _____.

31. Ms. Harold is incontinent. You help prevent UTIs by:

    A. _____

    B. _____

    C. _____

32. You are caring for an incontinent resident. You find yourself getting impatient. What should you do?

_____

33. List four reasons the doctor might order a catheter for a person.

    A. _____

    B. _____

    C. _____

    D. _____

34. Persons with catheters are at high risk for

_____.

35. You are giving catheter care. What observations do you need to report and record?

    A. _____

    B. _____

    C. _____

    D. _____

    E. _____

36. The urinary drainage bag is always kept

_____ the person's bladder.

37. What should you do if a urinary drainage system is accidentally disconnected?

    A. _____

       _____

    B. _____

       _____

    C. _____

       _____

    D. _____

       _____

    E. _____

       _____

    F. _____

       _____

    G. _____

       _____

38. A _____ is a soft,

rubber sheath that slides over the penis.

39. What is the goal of a bladder-training program?

_____

40. What information do you need from the nurse before collecting a urine specimen?

    A. _____

    B. _____

    C. _____

    D. _____

41. The _____ urine

specimen is collected for a urinalysis.

42. The midstream specimen is also called a

_____ or

_____.

43. Stools are normally _____,

_____, _____,

_____, and _____.

44. You must carefully observe stools before disposing of them. You need to observe and report the following:

    A. _____

    B. _____

    C. _____

    D. _____

    E. _____

    F. _____

45. List eight factors that affect the frequency, consistency, color, and odor of stools.

    A. _____

    B. _____

    C. _____

    D. _____

    E. _____

    F. _____

    G. _____

    H. _____

46. How does fluid intake affect bowel elimination?

    _____

    _____

    _____

    _____

47. Partially digested foods and fluids in the stomach are

    called _____.

48. Feces move through the intestines by

    _____.

49. _____ occurs

    when feces move slowly through the bowel.

50. Common causes of constipation include:

    A. _____

    B. _____

    C. _____

    D. _____

    E. _____

    F. _____

    G. _____

51. _____

    results if constipation is not relieved.

52. The nurse removes a fecal mass with a gloved finger.

    This is called _____

    _____.

53. Emotional effects of fecal incontinence include

    _____,

    _____,

    _____, and

    _____.

54. If flatus is not expelled, the intestines distend. List three measures that often produce flatus.

    A. _____

    B. _____

    C. _____

55. What are the two goals of bowel training?

    A. _____

    B. _____

56. A suppository is _____

_____

_____.

57. Why do doctors order enemas?

_____

_____

58. Enemas are dangerous for _____

_____

_____.

59. Stool consistency depends on the colostomy site. If a

colostomy is near the start of the colon, stools are

_____.

60. Ostomy pouch odors are prevented by:

A. _____

B. _____

C. _____

D. _____

61. Ms. Mann wears an ostomy pouch. You need to assist
with her tub bath. Why should you delay her bath for
1 to 2 hours after applying a new pouch?

_____

_____

62. What information do you need from the nurse before
collecting a stool specimen?

A. _____

B. _____

C. _____

Circle the BEST Answer

63. About how much urine does the healthy adult excrete
each day?
A. About 500 ml
B. About 1500 ml
C. About 3000 ml
D. About 700 ml

64. This is a bladder infection caused by bacteria.
A. Renal calculi
B. Pyelonephritis
C. Renal failure
D. Cystitis

65. Normal urine
A. Is pale yellow, straw colored, or amber
B. Does not have an odor
C. Is cloudy
D. Contains particles

66. You promote normal bladder elimination by
A. Setting new voiding routines
B. Asking the person to hurry
C. Providing only small amounts of fluid
D. Providing privacy

67. Which is *not* a nursing measure for persons with uri-
nary incontinence?
A. Increase fluid intake at bedtime.
B. Provide good skin care.
C. Answer signal lights promptly.
D. Encourage voiding at scheduled intervals.

68. You feel impatient when caring for a person with
incontinence. You must
A. Tell a co-worker to take care of the person for you.
B. Wait to provide care until you feel less stressed.
C. Discuss the problem with the nurse at once.
D. Refuse to care for the person.

69. Which statement about caring for persons with in-
dwelling catheters is *incorrect?*
A. Do not let the drainage bag rest on the floor.
B. Report leaks to the nurse at once.
C. Provide perineal care daily and after bowel
movements.
D. Attach the drainage bag to the bedrail.

70. When giving catheter care, you need to do all of the
following *except*
A. Check for crusts, abnormal drainage, or secretions.
B. Hold the catheter near the meatus.
C. Clean the catheter from the meatus down the
catheter about 4 inches.
D. Secure the catheter to the person's gown or
clothing.

71. When collecting specimens, you need to
    A. Use any available container.
    B. Label the container accurately.
    C. Collect the specimen whenever you have time.
    D. Ask the person to place the toilet paper in the specimen collection container.

72. Which statement about fecal incontinence is *incorrect?*
    A. A bowel-training program may be effective.
    B. Fecal incontinence affects the person emotionally.
    C. Fecal incontinence is always permanent.
    D. Fecal incontinence can result from unanswered signal lights.

73. Ms. Lopez has had a bowel movement. The stool is black in color and has a tarry consistency. You need to
    A. Ask Ms. Lopez if she has had anything unusual to eat.
    B. Ask the nurse to observe the stool.
    C. Dispose of the stool and report the color to the nurse.
    D. Ask a co-worker if this is normal for Ms. Lopez.

74. Which is *not* a cleansing enema?
    A. A small volume enema
    B. A soapsuds enema
    C. A tap-water enema
    D. A saline enema

75. Which measure does *not* promote comfort and safety when giving a small-volume enema to an adult?
    A. A comfortable right side-lying position
    B. Inserting the enema tip 2 inches into the rectum
    C. Stopping if the person complains of pain, you feel resistance, or bleeding occurs
    D. Placing the signal light and toilet tissue within reach

76. Liquid feces drain constantly from an ileostomy.
    A. True
    B. False

77. Used ostomy pouches are flushed down the toilet.
    A. True
    B. False

Additional Learning Activities

1. Think of your urination (voiding) patterns.
   A. List the factors that affect your daily patterns.

   B. Do changes in your patterns affect your comfort? Explain.

   C. Are you aware of how your diet, fluid intake, and level of activity affect your bowel elimination routines? Explain.

   D. Have you had personal experience with constipation or diarrhea? How did the experience affect your comfort?

2. Carefully review and practice the procedure for giving a bed pan. Work with a classmate. Use a regular bedpan and a fracture pan.
   A. Use the procedure checklist provided on pages 188-189 as a guide.
   B. Take your turn being the resident. Discuss your experience.
      (1) Did you have concerns about dignity and privacy?

(2) Was the experience physically comfortable? Explain.

(3) Was it difficult to position the bedpan correctly? Explain.

(4) Would you like to be left on a bedpan for 15 minutes or $1/2$ hour?

(5) How will your experience affect the care you give?

3. Do you know anyone with a colostomy or ileostomy? If the person is willing, discuss how the ostomy has affected his or her life. Ask these questions.
    A. How did the person adjust?

    B. What is the person's daily routine?

    C. How does the person care for the skin?

4. If available at your school or place of work, examine several types of colostomy and ileostomy pouches. Read the manufacturer's instructions. Practice handling the pouches and applying them on yourself and a willing classmate.

5. Handle the various types of enema equipment and become familiar with how each is used. This will increase your comfort and confidence.

6. Read the vignette; then answer the questions that follow.

    Mr. Chan is an 81-year-old resident of Pine Ridge Nursing Center. He has problems with constipation. He has not had a bowel movement for 4 days. He is complaining of abdominal discomfort. The nurse checked Mr. Chan for a fecal impaction. The doctor ordered a small-volume enema for Mr. Chan. The nurse delegated the procedure to you.

    A. What information do you need from the nurse before you give the enema?

    B. What items do you need to collect for the procedure?

    C. How will you explain the procedure to Mr. Chan?

    D. How will you provide for Mr. Chan's privacy?

    E. How will you provide for Mr. Chan's safety?

F. What observations do you need to report and
    record?

7. Carefully review all the procedures in Chapter 13.
    A. Under the supervision of your instructor, practice
        the procedures in Chapter 13. Use a simulator
        when appropriate. Use the procedure checklists
        provided on pages 188-204 as a guide.
    B. If any of these procedures embarrass you, discuss
        your feelings with your instructor.

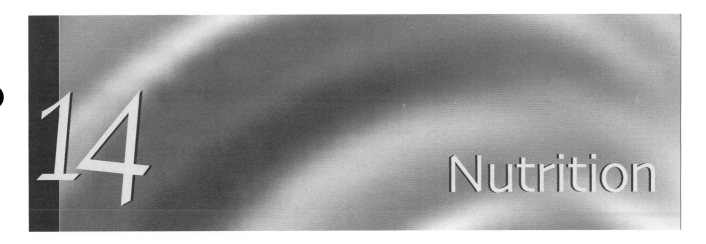

Nutrition

OBJECTIVES

The questions and student activities in this chapter will help you meet these objectives.
- Define the key terms listed in Chapter 14
- Explain the purpose and use of the Food Guide Pyramid
- Describe factors that affect eating and nutrition
- Describe the special diets
- Identify the signs, symptoms, and precautions relating to regurgitation and aspiration

- Describe fluid requirements and the causes of dehydration
- Explain what to do when the person has special fluid orders
- Explain how to assist with enteral nutrition and intravenous (IV) therapy
- Perform the procedures described in Chapter 14

Study Questions

Matching

Match each term with the correct definition.

1. _____ Loss of appetite

2. _____ Breathing fluid or an object into the lungs

3. _____ The amount of energy produced when the body burns food

4. _____ Difficulty swallowing

5. _____ Giving nutrients through the gastrointestinal tract

6. _____ Tube feeding

7 _____ A tube inserted through the nose into the stomach

8. _____ A substance that is ingested, digested, absorbed, and used by the body

9. _____ Giving fluids through a needle or catheter inserted into a vein

10. _____ The processes involved in the ingestion, digestion, absorption, and use of foods and fluids by the body

11. _____ The backward flow of food from the stomach into the mouth

12. _____ A decrease in the amount of water in body tissues

13. _____ The swelling of body tissues with water

A. IV therapy

B. Calorie

C. Nasogastric (NG) tube

D. Regurgitation

E. Dysphagia

F. Aspiration

G. Nutrient

H. Dehydration

I. Nutrition

J. Enteral nutrition

K. Gavage

L. Anorexia

M. Edema

Fill in the Blanks

14. The process of breaking down food physically and

    chemically for use by the cells is called

    _____.

15. The alimentary canal (GI tract) extends from the

    _____ to the

    _____.

16. Digestion begins in the _____

    _____.

17. _____ moistens

    food particles for easier swallowing and begins the

    digestion of food.

18. Involuntary muscle contractions called

    _____ move

    food down the esophagus into the stomach.

19. With diabetes, the body cannot produce or use

    _____ properly.

20. List five complications that can occur if diabetes is
    not controlled.

    A. _____

    B. _____

    C. _____

    D. _____

    E. _____

21. Which ethnic groups are at risk for Type 2 diabetes?

    A. _____

    B. _____

    C. _____

    D. _____

22. Type 1 diabetes is treated with

    _____,

    _____,

    and _____.

23. Both Type 1 and Type 2 diabetes require

    _____ monitoring.

24. _____

    means low sugar in the blood.

25. Nutrients are grouped into _____,

    _____, _____,

    _____, _____,

    and _____.

26. The amount of energy provided by nutrients is mea-

    sured in _____.

27. List the six food groups in the Food Guide Pyramid.

    A. _____

    B. _____

    C. _____

    D. _____

    E. _____

    F. _____

28. _____ provide

    energy and fiber for bowel elimination.

29. Minerals are needed for _____

    _____

    _____.

30. List six factors affecting eating and nutrition.

    A. _____

    B. _____

    C. _____

    D. _____

    E. _____

    F. _____

31. How does culture affect eating and nutrition?

    _____

    _____

32. Doctors order special diets for the following reasons:

    A. _____

    B. _____

33. _____ causes

    the body to retain water.

34. A diabetes meal plan developed by the dietitian and the person involves:

    A. _____

    _____

    B. _____

    _____

    C. _____

    _____

35. Mr. Jenkins has Type 1 diabetes. Why is it important to tell the nurse how much food he eats at each meal?

    _____

    _____

    _____

36. Which vitamins are not stored in the body?

    A. _____

    B. _____

37. Which diet involves changing food thickness to meet the person's needs?

    _____

38. You are assisting a person with dysphagia to eat. What observations do you need to report to the nurse at once?

    A. _____

    B. _____

    C. _____

    D. _____

39. Fluid balance is needed for health. The amount of

    fluid _____ and the

    amount of fluid _____

    must be equal.

40. How much fluid intake is needed per day for normal fluid balance?

    _____

41. Encourage fluids means _____

    _____

    _____

    _____.

42. NPO is an abbreviation for _____

    _____.

43. Ms. Mann's meal tray has been sitting on a cart outside her room for 25 minutes. What should you do?

_____

_____

44. What information do you need from the nurse and the care plan before serving meal trays?

A. _____

B. _____

C. _____

45. Why are spoons used to feed people?

_____

46. How do you help a visually impaired person locate food on the tray?

_____

_____

47. Where should you position yourself to feed a person?

_____

48. You are feeding Ms. Sanchez. What observations do you need to report and record?

A. _____

B. _____

C. _____

D. _____

49. Ms. Sanchez has water, milk, and coffee on her tray. How many straws should be on the tray?

_____

_____

50. When are between-meal nourishments served?

_____

51. A _____ is inserted into the stomach through a surgically created opening.

52. _____ is a major risk of enteral nutrition.

53. Which health team member is responsible for checking tube placement before a feeding?

_____

54. Doctors order IV therapy to:

A. _____

B. _____

C. _____

D. _____

E. _____

55. Ms. Omar is receiving IV therapy. An electronic pump is being used. The pump alarms while you are taking Ms. Omar's vital signs. What should you do?

_____

Circle the BEST Answer

56. Which statement about age-related changes in the GI tract is *false?*
    A. Salivary glands produce less saliva.
    B. Secretion of digestive juices decreases.
    C. More calories are needed.
    D. Peristalsis decreases.

57. Which type of diabetes has a rapid onset and occurs in children and young adults?
    A. Type 1
    B. Type 2
    C. Gestational diabetes
    D. Combination diabetes

58. Which is *not* a sign of hyperglycemia?
    A. Drowsiness
    B. Restlessness and agitation
    C. Sweet breath odor
    D. Frequent urination

59. Which are signs and symptoms of hypoglycemia?
    A. Sweating, headache, dizziness, and rapid pulse
    B. High blood pressure, frequent urination, and chest pain
    C. Loss of appetite and slow and deep respirations
    D. High blood pressure; slow pulse; and warm, dry skin

60. The Food Guide Pyramid encourages
    A. A high fat diet
    B. Eating a variety of foods
    C. A diet high in sodium
    D. Eating only small amounts of fruits and vegetables

61. How many servings from the vegetable group are recommended daily?
    A. 1-2 servings
    B. 5-7 servings
    C. 3-5 servings
    D. 7-9 servings

62. The meat, poultry, fish, dry beans, eggs, and nuts group
    A. Is lower in fat than the milk, yogurt, and cheese group
    B. Contains some sugar
    C. Is high in fiber, vitamin E, and minerals
    D. Is high in protein and fat

63. Protein is an important nutrient because
    A. It provides fiber for bowel elimination.
    B. It is needed for tissue growth and repair.
    C. It helps the body use certain vitamins.
    D. It does not provide calories.

64. How many calories are in one gram of fat?
    A. 4 calories
    B. 6 calories
    C. 9 calories
    D. 12 calories

65. Which is *not* an OBRA requirement for food served in nursing centers?
    A. The person's diet is well balanced and nourishing.
    B. Hot food is served hot. Cold food is served cold.
    C. Each person receives at least three snacks each day.
    D. The center provides any special eating equipment.

66. To prepare a person for meals, you need the following information *except*
    A. How much help the person needs
    B. The person's gender
    C. Where the person will eat
    D. How to position the person

67. Which action will *not* prevent the spread of infection when providing drinking water?
    A. Making sure the water pitcher is labeled with person's name and room and bed number
    B. Not touching the rim or inside of the water glass or pitcher
    C. Not letting the ice scoop touch the rim or inside of the water glass or pitcher
    D. Placing the ice scoop inside the ice container or dispenser

68. Diabetes is a chronic disease from lack of insulin. Insulin allows the body to use
    A. Sugar
    B. Fat
    C. Protein
    D. Minerals

69. When feeding a person
    A. Always use a fork.
    B. Stand facing the person.
    C. Ask the person about the order in which to offer food and fluids.
    D. Encourage the person to take liquids after every bite.

70. Mr. Paul is receiving a tube feeding. To prevent regurgitation and aspiration, you need to
    A. Provide frequent oral hygiene.
    B. Position him in the left side-lying position for the tube feeding.
    C. Give formula rapidly.
    D. Position him in the semi-Fowler's position during and after the tube feeding.

71. NPO is ordered for Mr. Nunn. This means
    A. Fluid intake is increased.
    B. He cannot eat or drink anything.
    C. Water is offered in small amounts.
    D. Fluids are restricted.

72. Your role in caring for persons receiving IV therapy includes
    A. Meeting hygiene and activity needs
    B. Regulating the flow rate
    C. Changing IV bags
    D. Adding drugs to IV solutions

73. Which food is *not* allowed on a clear liquid diet?
    A. Water
    B. Tea
    C. Apple juice
    D. Ice cream

74. Ms. Parker eats slowly. She frequently coughs while eating and complains that food will not go down. These are signs and symptoms of
    A. Diabetes
    B. Dysphagia
    C. Dementia
    D. Pneumonia

75. Which of the following is a safety measure for IV therapy?
    A. Follow clean technique.
    B. Remove the IV bag when assisting the person with ambulation.
    C. Always allow enough slack on the IV tubing when moving or turning the person in bed.
    D. Keep the person in bed, and restrain the arm with the IV.

Additional Learning Activities

1. Discuss the importance of food in your life. Answer these questions.
   A. Besides meeting physical needs, what role does food play in your life?

   B. Do your cultural background and religious beliefs affect which foods you eat and how you prepare your food? Explain.

   C. What role does food play in your social life?

2. Has illness ever affected your appetite or your ability to eat certain foods?

   A. How might your experience affect the care you provide?

3. Review the Food Guide Pyramid (page 268 in the textbook).
   A. Are you making wise food choices? Explain.

   B. Is your diet well balanced? Explain.

4. List the age-related changes in the digestive system. Discuss how these changes affect:
   A. What the person eats

   B. How the person prepares food

   C. The person's enjoyment of food

5. Carefully review the procedures for serving meal trays and feeding a person.
   A. Use the procedure checklists on pages 205-209 as a guide.
   B. Practice the procedures with a classmate using various food consistencies.
   C. Take your turn being the resident. Discuss your experience. Answer these questions:
      (1) How does it feel to be fed by another person?

      (2) Did you enjoy your meal? Explain.

      (3) Were you fed too fast or too slow?

   (4) Was the amount given with each bite right for you?

   (5) Were liquids offered during the meal?

   (6) Did your food remain at the right temperature throughout the meal?

   (7) How might your experience affect the care you give?

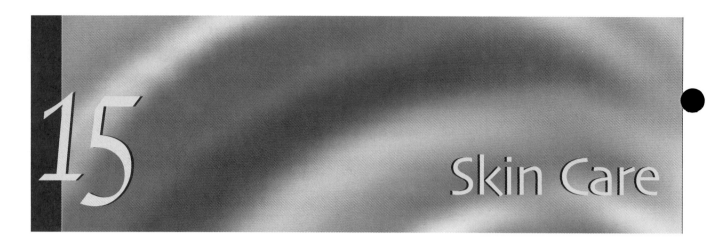

15 Skin Care

OBJECTIVES

The questions and student activities in this chapter will help you meet these objectives.
- Define the key terms listed in Chapter 15
- Describe skin tears and how to prevent them
- Describe pressure ulcers and how to prevent them
- Identify the pressure points in each body position
- Describe circulatory ulcers and how to prevent them
- Explain the purpose of elastic stockings
- Perform the procedure described in Chapter 15

Study Questions

Matching

Match each term with the correct definition.

1. _____ The rubbing of one surface against another

2. _____ A condition in which there is death of tissue

3. _____ A blood clot

4. _____ When the skin sticks to a surface while muscles slide in the direction the body is moving

5. _____ Open wounds on the lower legs and feet caused by poor blood return from veins

6. _____ A break in the skin or mucous membrane

7. _____ A break or rip in the skin; the epidermis separates from the underlying tissues

8. _____ An open wound on the lower legs and feet caused by decreased blood flow through the arteries or veins; vascular ulcer

9. _____ Any injury caused by unrelieved pressure

10. _____ A pressure ulcer, pressure sore, or bedsore

A. Shearing

B. Circulatory ulcer

C. Pressure ulcer

D. Friction

E. Skin tear

F. Decubitus ulcer

G. Gangrene

H. Wound

I. Stasis ulcer

J. Thrombus

Fill in the Blanks

11. List four causes of skin tears.

    A. _____

    B. _____

    C. _____

    D. _____

12. The _____,

    _____,

    and _____

    are common sites for skin tears.

13. Older and disabled persons are at great risk for pressure ulcers because of:

    A. _____

    B. _____

    C. _____

14. Persons at risk for pressure ulcers are those who:

    A. _____

    B. _____

    C. _____

    D. _____

    E. _____

    F. _____

    G. _____

    H. _____

15. The first sign of a pressure ulcer is _____

    _____

    _____.

16. Pressure ulcers occur over bony areas. The bony

    areas are called _____.

17. What is the purpose of a bed cradle?

    _____

    _____

18. Arterial ulcers are

    _____

    _____

    _____.

19. Elastic stockings are often ordered to promote

    _____.

20. When are elastic stockings applied?

    _____

21. What information do you need from the nurse and the care plan before applying elastic stockings?

    A. _____

    B. _____

    C. _____

    D. _____

22. Why do you need to make sure elastic stockings do not have twists, creases, or wrinkles after you apply them?

    _____

    _____

    _____

Circle the BEST Answer

23. To prevent skin tears you need to do all of the following *except*
    A. Keep your fingernails short and smoothly filed.
    B. Report long and tough toenails to the nurse.
    C. Dress the person in short-sleeved clothing with zippers.
    D. Use a lift sheet to lift and turn the person in bed.

24. Mr. Quinn has a stage 2 pressure ulcer. This means
    A. The skin is red and intact.
    B. The skin cracks, blisters, or peels. There may be a shallow crater.
    C. The skin is gone. Underlying tissues are exposed. There may be drainage.
    D. Muscle and bone are exposed and damaged. Drainage is likely.

25. Which measure will help prevent pressure ulcers?
    A. Follow the repositioning schedule in the person's care plan.
    B. When the person is in bed, raise the head of the bed 45 degrees.
    C. Scrub the skin vigorously when bathing and drying the person.
    D. Always use soap when bathing the person.

26. Ms. Romero sits in her wheelchair most of the day. How often does she need to shift positions?
    A. Every 2 hours
    B. Whenever she thinks about it
    C. Every hour
    D. Every 15 minutes

27. Which measure will *not* help prevent circulatory ulcers?
    A. Keeping the feet clean and dry
    B. Making sure shoes fit well
    C. Having the person use rubber band type garters to hold socks or hose in place
    D. Keeping pressure off the heels and other bony areas

28. Common sites for arterial ulcers are
    A. On the lower arms and the hands
    B. On the buttocks, back, and shoulders
    C. Between abdominal folds and under the breasts
    D. Between the toes, on top of the toes, and on the outer side of the ankles

29. How often are elastic stockings removed?
    A. Every 8 hours or according to the care plan
    B. Every morning before breakfast
    C. As often as the person requests
    D. Whenever the person gets out of bed

30. You must never rub or massage reddened areas.
    A. True
    B. False

Labeling

31. Place an *X* on each of the pressure points in the following drawings.

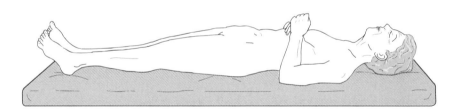

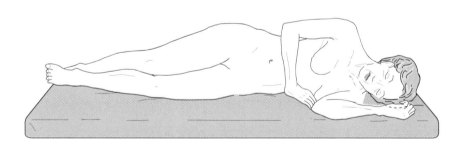

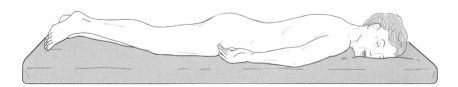

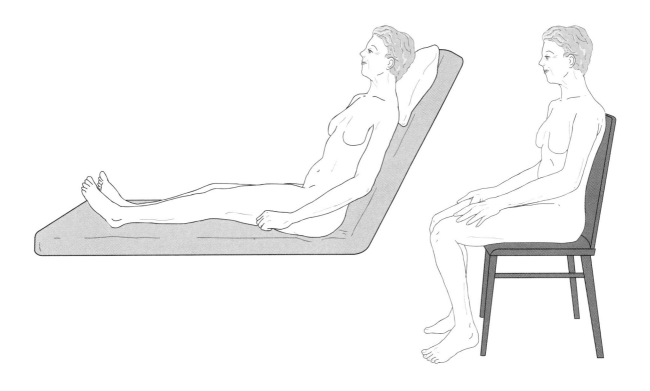

Additional Learning Activities

1. Sit in a hard, straight-backed chair for 20 minutes. Do not shift your position. Notice any pressure area. Notice changes in your comfort level. Think of how it would feel to be in a chair for 2 hours or more without being able to change positions or get up and walk around.

2. Lay in bed in a side-lying position for 20 minutes. Do not change your position. Notice pressure areas. Notice changes in your comfort level. Think about how you would feel if you were unable to change your position for 2 hours or longer.

3. Under the supervision of your instructor, practice the procedure in Chapter 15. Use the procedure checklist on page 210 as a guide. Take your turn being the resident.

16 Assisting With Moving and Positioning

OBJECTIVES

The questions and student activities in this chapter will help you meet these objectives.
- Define the key terms listed in Chapter 16
- Identify comfort and safety measures for lifting, turning, and moving persons in bed
- Explain the purpose of a transfer belt (gait belt)
- Explain how to safely perform transfer procedures
- Explain why body alignment and position changes are important
- Identify the comfort and safety measures for positioning a person
- Position persons in the basic bed positions and in a chair
- Perform the procedures described in Chapter 16

Study Questions

Matching

Match each term with the correct definition.

1. _____ Lying on the abdomen with the head turned to one side

2. _____ The back-lying or dorsal recumbent position

3. _____ A cotton draw sheet that is used to move the person in bed and reduce friction; turning sheet

4. _____ Turning the person as a unit, in alignment, with one motion

5. _____ A belt used to support persons who are unsteady or disabled; gait belt

6. _____ A left side-lying position in which the upper leg is sharply flexed so it is not on the lower leg and the lower arm is behind the person

7. _____ The side-lying position

A. Lateral position

B. Prone position

C. Transfer belt

D. Logrolling

E. Supine position

F. Sims' position

G. Lift sheet

Fill in the Blanks

8. Why is it important to use good body mechanics when moving and positioning persons?

   _____

   _____

9. Friction and shearing injure the skin. They both cause

   _____ and

   _____.

10. You reduce friction and shearing by

    _____ or _____

    the person.

11. For safety and efficiency, when do you need to decide how you will move the person?

_____

12. Why are beds raised horizontally to lift and move persons in bed?

_____

_____

13. At least two workers are needed to move

_____, _____,

and _____

persons up in bed.

14. After lifting or moving a person, you need to

_____.

15. You are getting ready to move Mr. Stevens up in bed. Why should you place the pillow against the headboard?

_____

_____

_____

16. Explain how you should stand when moving the person up in bed.

_____

_____

_____

17. You and co-worker are moving Mr. Thomas up in bed using a lift sheet. Where is the lift sheet placed?

_____

_____

18. Lift sheets are used to move the following persons up in bed:

A. _____

B. _____

C. _____

D. _____

19. You are preparing to turn Mr. Thomas from his left side to his right side. Why do you need to move him to the side of the bed before turning him?

_____

_____

20. You are moving Mr. Walters to the side of the bed in segments. Which part of his body should you move first?

_____

21. What information do you need from the nurse and the care plan before turning and repositioning a person?

A. _____

_____

B. _____

_____

C. _____

_____

D. _____

_____

E. _____

_____

F. _____

_____

22. Placing the person in good alignment helps prevent

_____,

_____, and

_____.

23. Logrolling is used to turn the following persons:

A. _____

B. _____

C. _____

D. _____

24. How many staff members are needed to logroll a person?

_____

25. To logroll a person, the bed is _____

_____.

26. You are assisting Ms. Young to dangle. She complains of feeling dizzy. What should you do?

_____

27. To transfer a person means _____

_____

_____.

28. Why do you need to know about areas of weakness before you transfer a person?

_____

_____

_____

_____

29. What observations do you need to report and record after transferring a person?

A. _____

_____

B. _____

_____

C. _____

_____

D. _____

_____

30. The person wears _____

footwear for transfers.

31. To prevent falls and injuries, bed wheels must be

_____ for transfers.

32. To use a transfer belt safely, you must always

_____.

33. If a person cannot assist with a chair, wheelchair, commode, or shower chair transfer, a

_____ is used.

34. Mr. Arnold is weak on his right side. On which side will you help him out of bed?

_____

35. The number of persons needed for a transfer depends on the person's _____,

_____, and

_____.

36. Before using a mechanical lift, you need to:

    A. _____
       _____

    B. _____
       _____

    C. _____
       _____

    D. _____
       _____

37. How is the wheelchair positioned for wheelchair to toilet transfers?

    _____
    _____
    _____
    _____

38. Whenever you reposition a person, make sure linens

    are _____ ,
    _____ , and
    _____ .

39. A contracture is _____
    _____
    _____
    _____ .

40. Contractures can develop from _____
    _____
    _____ .

41. You have positioned Ms. Barnett in Fowler's position. For good alignment, you must:

    A. _____

    B. _____

    C. _____

42. You have positioned Mr. Carson in the prone position. Where should you place pillows?

    _____
    _____

43. For good alignment, how should you position a person in the chair?

    A. _____
       _____

    B. _____
       _____

    C. _____
       _____

Circle the BEST Answer.

44. Ms. Vance is 90 years old and has arthritis. Before turning her, you need to move her to the side of the bed. You need to move her in segments.
    A. True
    B. False

45. You are helping Ms. Young to dangle. Which is *incorrect?*
    A. Provide support if necessary.
    B. Ask her how she feels.
    C. Check her pulse and respirations.
    D. Leave her alone if she tells you she is OK.

46. Transfer belts are always applied over clothing.
    A. True
    B. False

47. You are applying a transfer belt on Ms. Perez. Which is *incorrect?*
    A. The belt should be snug, but should not cause discomfort or impair breathing.
    B. You should be able to slide your open, flat hand under the belt.
    C. Make sure her breasts are not caught under the belt.
    D. Place the buckle in back over her spine.

48. You are transferring Ms. Reed from the bed to a wheelchair. Which is *correct?*
    A. Wheelchair wheels are unlocked for a safe transfer.
    B. She should support herself by putting her arms around your neck.
    C. After the transfer, position the wheelchair as she prefers.
    D. After positioning the wheelchair, always lock the wheels.

49. To position a person safely, you need to do all of the following *except*
    A. Use good body mechanics.
    B. Explain the procedure to the person.
    C. Position the person as quickly as possible.
    D. Place the signal light within reach after positioning.

50. Mr. Darby has a belt restraint when he sits in the chair. A pillow should be placed behind his back for comfort.
    A. True
    B. False

51. You are repositioning Mr. Green in the wheelchair. He is able to assist. Which is *correct?*
    A. Lock the wheelchair wheels.
    B. Stand behind him.
    C. Ask him to place his folded hands in his lap.
    D. Position his feet on the footplates.

52. You and a co-worker are repositioning Ms. Howard in her wheelchair. She cannot assist. The tallest worker stands in front of the wheelchair.
    A. True
    B. False

Additional Learning Activities

1. List the measures needed for good alignment for each of the following positions:
   A. Fowler's position

   B. Supine position

   C. Lateral position

   D. Sims' position

   E. Chair position

2. Describe how you would reposition a person in the chair or wheelchair:
   A. If the person is alert, cooperative, can follow instructions, and has the strength to help

B. If the person cannot assist with repositioning

b. Did you feel comfortable? Explain.

3. Review the procedures in Chapter 16.
   A. Under the supervision of your instructor, practice each procedure.
      (1) Use the procedure checklists provided on pages 211-231.
      (2) Take your turn being the resident.
      (3) Discuss the experience with your classmates and instructor. Answer these questions.

      a. Did you feel safe? Explain.

4. Practice proper positioning (Fowler's, supine, prone, lateral, and Sims') with a classmate or family member. Use pillows to promote comfort and good body alignment. Assume each position yourself.

17 Mental Health Needs

OBJECTIVES

The questions and student activities in this chapter will help you meet these objectives.
- Define the key terms listed in Chapter 17
- Identify the development tasks for each age-group
- Describe common reactions to the need for nursing center care
- Describe the psychological and social changes that occur with aging
- Describe the common reactions to aging and loss
- Explain how to deal with anger and other behavior issues
- Describe the common mental health disorders

Study Questions

Matching

Match each term with the correct definition.

1. _____ The person copes with and adjusts to everyday stresses in ways accepted by society

2. _____ Unconscious reactions that block unpleasant or threatening feelings

3. _____ A vague, uneasy feeling in response to stress

4. _____ Changes in mental, emotional, and social function

5. _____ A disturbance in the ability to cope with or adjust to stress

6. _____ The physical changes that are measured and that occur in a steady and orderly manner

7. _____ A skill that must be completed during a stage of development

A. Anxiety

B. Mental health

C. Development

D. Defense mechanism

E. Developmental task

F. Mental illness

G. Growth

Fill in the Blanks

8. Mental relates to _____

   _____.

9. Growth and development occur in a

   _____,

   _____,

   and _____.

10. List the developmental tasks of late adulthood (65 years and older).

    A. _____

    B. _____

    C. _____

    D. _____

    E. _____

11. _____ is a

common response to needing nursing center care.

12. Persons needing nursing center care may experience some or all of the following losses:

A. _____

B. _____

C. _____

D. _____

E. _____

13. Mr. Jones is a resident of Ocean View Nursing Center

because of increased difficulty with ambulation and

mild confusion. The health team focuses on

_____

_____.

You must help him _____

_____

_____.

14. Losses may cause the person to feel

_____, _____,

and _____.

15. How a person copes with aging depends on:

A. _____

B. _____

C. _____

D. _____

E. _____

16. When a person's partner dies, the person loses a

_____,

_____,

_____, and

_____.

17. _____ and

_____ are

used to relieve anxiety.

18. Describe the following behaviors:

A. Self-centered behavior

_____

_____

_____

B. Withdrawal

_____

_____

_____

19. Causes of demanding behavior include:

A. _____

B. _____

C. _____

D. _____

20. Some people have inappropriate sexual behaviors. List five possible causes for such behaviors.

A. _____

B. _____

C. _____

D. _____

E. _____

21. An obsession is _____
    _____.

22. _____ means split
    mind. It is a severe, chronic, disabling brain disease.

23. The person with bipolar disorder has
    _____
    _____.

24. Personality disorders involve _____
    and _____ behaviors.

25. Describe an antisocial personality.
    _____
    _____
    _____
    _____

26. Ms. Green has an abusive personality. This means
    _____
    _____
    _____.

27. Substance abuse occurs when _____
    _____
    _____
    _____.

28. List five causes of mental health disorders.

    A. _____

    B. _____

    C. _____

    D. _____

    E. _____

29. Mr. Hein was born in Russia. He does not understand or speak English well. There are no other Russian-speaking residents in the nursing center. Explain how Mr. Hein might feel.
    _____
    _____
    _____
    _____

30. Which defense mechanism is the person using in each of the following situations?
    A. A man has emphysema. He continues to smoke even though the doctor told him he would die if he did not stop smoking.
       _____

    B. Mary is late for school because she forgot to set her alarm and overslept. She blames her mother for not waking her.
       _____

    C. A 14-year-old girl starts sucking her thumb when her parents get a divorce.
       _____

Circle the BEST Answer

31. Retirement usually means
    A. Moving to a nursing center
    B. Reduced income
    C. Increased income
    D. Moving in with adult children

32. Which is *not* a development task of infancy?
    A. Learning to walk
    B. Learning to eat solid foods
    C. Developing stable sleep and feeding patterns
    D. Gaining control of bowel and bladder function

33. Which is a developmental task of adolescence?
    A. Developing a conscience and morals
    B. Learning how to study
    C. Becoming independent from parents and adults
    D. Adjusting to aging parents

34. Social relationships stay the same throughout life.
    A. True
    B. False

35. Ms. Ortega is 85 years old. She recently moved in with her adult daughter and her family. Which statement is *true?*
    A. Ms. Ortega will feel useless as long as she lives in her daughter's home.
    B. Ms. Ortega's daughter needs to place her mother in a nursing center.
    C. Everyone in the home will feel good about the situation.
    D. Everyone in the home will need to adjust.

36. Mr. Miles is a nursing center resident. He is angry because he had to give up his home and because he needs to depend on others to meet some of his basic needs. Which statement is *true?*
    A. Mr. Miles may show his anger verbally and nonverbally.
    B. You should avoid Mr. Miles when he is angry.
    C. You need to tell Mr. Miles that being angry will not help him.
    D. If you ignore Mr. Miles, he will get over being angry.

37. Some anxiety is normal.
    A. True
    B. False

38. Ms. Roberts is critical of others. Nothing seems to please her. She wants things done at the same time every day. This is
    A. Dementia
    B. Angry behavior
    C. Aggressive behavior
    D. Demanding behavior

39. Ms. Miles yells at you when you try to help her. She tells you that you do not know how to take care of her. You can do all of the following *except*
    A. Answer her questions clearly and thoroughly.
    B. Stay calm and professional.
    C. Argue with her and let her know that you do know how to care for her.
    D. Answer her signal light promptly.

40. Mr. Lyons is angry. He is shouting and becoming more agitated. You should do all of the following *except*
    A. Stand close to him and use touch to calm him.
    B. Stand close to the door.
    C. Keep your hands free.
    D. Leave the room as soon as you can.

41. Which defense mechanism means refusing to accept or believe something that is true?
    A. Compensation
    B. Projection
    C. Rationalization
    D. Denial

42. Ms. Granger is angry with her son because he does not visit her. She yells at you when you enter her room. Which defense mechanism is she using?
    A. Displacement
    B. Regression
    C. Repression
    D. Compensation

43. Mr. Ryan believes that his roommate is a foreign spy. This is a
    A. Hallucination
    B. Depressive illness
    C. Delusion
    D. Psychosis

44. To adapt means to
    A. Change or adjust
    B. Be rigid
    C. Lack morals
    D. Blame others for one's actions

45. Depression is common in older persons
    A. True
    B. False

46. Dependence on drugs or alcohol can be emotional, psychological, or physical.
    A. True
    B. False

47. Which is *not* a sign or symptom of depression?
    A. Agitation
    B. Fatigue
    C. High energy level
    D. Feelings of helplessness

Additional Learning Activities

1. Ask an older relative, friend, or neighbor if you can interview him or her. Ask the person:
   A. What physical, social, and psychological changes has he or she experienced over the past 10 to 20 years?

   B. How has the person adjusted?

   C. What changes have been most difficult to cope with? Why?

   D. Who provides support for the person?

   E. What concerns does the person have about the future?

   F. What things bring joy and meaning to the person's life?

2. Carefully read about the changes that occur as people age. Think about how these changes might affect you and your life-style as you age. Answer these questions:
   A. What are your fears and concerns?

   B. How do you plan to adjust to the changes?

   C. What people and possessions might you have the most difficulty giving up? Explain.

3. Review the developmental tasks of your age-group.
   A. Describe the tasks that have meaning to you.

   B. What are some ways you are involved in completing each task?

   C. What developmental tasks are other members of your family involved in completing?

4. Interview a person who has recently retired. Ask the person to discuss how retirement has affected his or her life-style.

5. Write down how you are preparing for retirement financially, socially, and physically.

6. Think of stresses in your personal life that cause you to feel anxious.
   A. How do you feel when you are anxious?

B. What defense mechanisms do you use to cope with anxiety?

7. Do you have personal fears about caring for persons with mental health problems? Explain.

A. How might your feelings and fears affect the care you provide?

B. How might you handle your fears so that you are able to provide quality care?

18 Care of Cognitively Impaired Residents

OBJECTIVES

The questions and student activities in this chapter will help you meet these objectives.
- Define the key terms listed in Chapter 18
- Describe confusion, its causes, and related care measures
- Explain the difference between delirium, depression, and dementia
- Describe Alzheimer's disease (AD) and its signs, symptoms, and behaviors
- Explain the care required by persons with AD and other dementias
- Describe the effects of AD on the family

Study Questions

Matching

Match each term with the correct definition.

1. _____ A state of temporary but acute mental confusion

2. _____ A false belief

3. _____ Extreme responses; person reacts as if there is a disaster or tragedy

4. _____ Seeing, hearing, or feeling something that is not real

5. _____ Signs, symptoms, and behaviors of AD increase during hours of darkness

6. _____ The loss of cognitive and social function caused by changes in the brain

7. _____ Dementia caused by many strokes

A. Catastrophic reactions

B. Dementia

C. Multi-infarct dementia

D. Delirium

E. Sundowning

F. Hallucination

G. Delusion

Fill in the Blanks

8. Cognitive functioning involves:

   A. _____

   B. _____

   C. _____

   D. _____

   E. _____

   F. _____

9. List five causes of acute confusion.

   A. _____

   B. _____

   C. _____

   D. _____

   E. _____

10. Treatment of delirium is aimed at

_____.

11. Mr. Jones is confused. List four measures that might help him maintain the day night cycle.

    A. _____

    B. _____

    C. _____

    D. _____

12. _____ is the

most common type of permanent dementia.

13. List four treatable causes of dementia.

    A. _____

    B. _____

    C. _____

    D. _____

14. Signs and symptoms of delirium include:

    A. _____

    B. _____

    C. _____

    D. _____

    E. _____

    F. _____

    G. _____

    H. _____

15. Explain why depression is often overlooked in older persons.

    _____

    _____

16. The classic sign of AD is _____

_____.

17. What is the purpose of the "Safe Return Program" sponsored by the Alzheimer's Association?

    _____

    _____

18. Catastrophic reactions are common from

    _____.

19. How might you cause a person with AD to become agitated?

    _____

    _____

20. Sexual behaviors are labeled abnormal because of

    _____

    _____.

21. Abnormal sexual behaviors may involve:

    A. _____

    B. _____

    C. _____

22. List four nonsexual reasons that a person with AD may touch, scratch, or rub his or her genitals.

    A. _____

    B. _____

    C. _____

    D. _____

23. Mr. John Kane has AD. He is a resident at Valley View Nursing Center. Why is it important to report any changes in his usual behavior to the nurse?

    _____

    _____

24. Therapists often work with persons with AD. Therapies and activities focus on _____

_____.

25. Persons in the early stages of AD often live at home with family. Long-term care is needed when:

A. _____

B. _____

C. _____

D. _____

E. _____

F. _____

26. Often adult children are caught in the *sandwich generation*. What does this mean?

_____

_____

27. What is the purpose of Alzheimer's support groups?

_____

_____

_____

28. List three measures that will protect the person's right to privacy and confidentiality.

A. _____

_____

B. _____

_____

C. _____

_____

Circle the BEST Answer

29. Which is *not* a change in the nervous system from aging?
    A. Brain cells are lost.
    B. Response and reaction times are slower.
    C. Touch and sensitivity to pain increase.
    D. Changes in sleep patterns occur.

30. Confusion caused by physical changes cannot be cured.
    A. True
    B. False

31. Mr. Jones is confused. Which of the following measures will *not* help improve function?
    A. Face him and speak clearly and slowly.
    B. Change his schedule every day.
    C. Tell him what you are going to do and why.
    D. Tell him the date and time each morning.

32. Which is an *early* warning sign of dementia?
    A. Recent memory loss that affects job skills
    B. Movement and gait problems
    C. Fecal incontinence
    D. The person does not recognize family members.

33. The most common mental health problem in older persons is
    A. Delirium
    B. Anxiety
    C. Depression
    D. Bi-polar disorder

34. Ms. Adams has AD. You know that
    A. The onset is sudden.
    B. AD usually occurs before the age of 65.
    C. Men are affected more often than women.
    D. The cause is unknown.

35. A person in stage 1 of AD may have the following signs and symptoms
    A. Restlessness, sleep problems, and fecal and urinary incontinence
    B. Agitation, delusions, and problems communicating
    C. Memory loss, disorientation to time and place, and moodiness
    D. Seizures, dysphagia, and coma

36. Mr. Gomez has AD. He frequently wanders into other resident rooms. You know that
    A. Wandering always has a cause.
    B. You must keep him confined to his room.
    C. He wants to take things from other resident rooms.
    D. Pain, drug side effects, stress, and anxiety are possible causes.

37. Ms. Adams has AD. You promote her safety by
    A. Keeping her restrained
    B. Explaining safety rules to her
    C. Changing her room frequently
    D. Keeping noise levels low

38. Persons with AD may scream to communicate.
    A. True
    B. False

39. Ms. Adams has AD. She is walking in the hallway and screaming. You can help by
    A. Calmly asking her to stop
    B. Taking her to her room and closing the door
    C. Turning on loud music
    D. Using touch to calm her

40. Mr. Gomez is masturbating in the dining room. What should you do?
    A. Tell him that his behavior is bad and take him to his room.
    B. Ignore his behavior.
    C. Tell his family about the behavior when they visit.
    D. Lead him to his room. Provide privacy and safety.

41. Repetitive behaviors usually are harmful to the person.
    A. True
    B. False

42. The person with AD
    A. Chooses to be incontinent
    B. Needs your support and understanding
    C. Has control over his or her actions
    D. Can understand and follow instructions

43. Restraints can make confusion and demented behaviors worse.
    A. True
    B. False

44. You are helping Ms. Adams with dressing and grooming. She is agitated and trying to hit you. You find yourself feeling frustrated and impatient. What should you do?
    A. Leave the room and come back later.
    B. Tell a co-worker to finish dressing and grooming Ms. Adams.
    C. Talk to the nurse.
    D. Call Ms. Adams' daughter.

45. Proper use of validation therapy requires special training.
    A. True
    B. False

46. Which statement about family members of person's with AD is *false?*
    A. They often feel helpless.
    B. Guilt feelings are common.
    C. They help plan care whenever possible.
    D. You do not need to be concerned with the needs of family members.

Additional Learning Activities

1. If you can, talk to a family member of someone with AD:
   A. Discuss the effects of the disease on the family. Ask the following questions.
      (1) What were the first signs and symptoms noticed by the family?

      (2) Is the person cared for in the home?

      (3) What support systems are in place?

      (4) If the person is in a nursing center, how do members of the health care team provide care?

2. Compare the signs and symptoms of delirium, depression, and early AD. Answer the following questions:

   A. How are the signs and symptoms similar?

   B. Why is it important to have a correct diagnosis?

3. Read the vignette; then answer the questions that follow.

Ms. Lynn Abbott has AD. She has been living in her daughter's home. Her daughter works full time. She was able to meet her mother's needs with the following in-home services:

- *A home care aide to assist with Ms. Abbott's bath twice a week*
- *Her mother attends an adult day-care program 3 days a week.*
- *A volunteer from Ms. Abbott's church visits 1 day a week.*
- *Ms. Abbott and her daughter belong to an Alzheimer's support group.*

During the past 2 weeks, Ms. Abbott has left her daughter's home three times. Twice a neighbor brought her home, and once she was found wandering in a grocery store five blocks from her daughter's home. Often Ms. Abbott refuses to get dressed in the morning. She has also been incontinent of bladder several times in the past few days. She is becoming less interested in her personal hygiene. She has started to resist her daughter's efforts to bathe her. Ms. Abbott's daughter is afraid to leave her alone for even short periods of time. When Ms. Abbott is not at the adult day-care program, her daughter comes home during her lunch hour to check on her. If her daughter wants to go out in the evening, she gets a sitter to stay with Ms. Abbott. She is looking for a nursing center for her mother. This is very difficult, as she feels she should care for her mother herself.

A. What behaviors might be causing Ms. Abbott's daughter to consider placement in a nursing center?

B. What health and safety risks does Ms. Abbott have?

C. What effect does Ms. Abbott's AD have on her daughter's daily life?

D. What financial impact does Ms. Abbott's AD have?

E. What support systems is Ms. Abbott's daughter using?

F. What physical needs does Ms. Abbott have? Are Ms. Abbott's physical needs likely to increase? Explain.

G. What psychosocial needs does Ms. Abbott have? Are her psychosocial needs likely to increase? Explain.

I. What fears might Ms. Abbott's daughter have about placing her mother in a nursing center?

H. What needs might Ms. Abbott's daughter have?

19 Basic Restorative Care

OBJECTIVES

The questions and student activities in this chapter will help you meet these objectives.
- Define the key terms listed in Chapter 19
- Describe how aging and common health problems affect the nervous system
- Describe how rehabilitation and restorative care involve the whole person
- Identify the complications to prevent
- Describe the physical, psychological, and social aspects of rehabilitation and restorative care
- Describe common self-help and positioning devices
- Explain the rules for performing range-of-motion exercises
- Describe four walking aids
- Explain your role in rehabilitation and restorative care
- Explain how to promote quality of life
- Perform the procedures described in Chapter 19

Study Questions

Matching

Match each term with the correct definition.

1. _____ The decrease in size or a wasting away of tissue

2. _____ Any lost, absent, or impaired physical or mental function

3. _____ An artificial replacement for a missing body part

4. _____ The activities usually done during a normal day in a person's life

5. _____ The process of restoring the person to the highest possible level of physical, psychological, social, and economic function

6. _____ Care that helps persons regain their health, strength, and independence

7. _____ A nursing assistant with special training in restorative nursing and rehabilitation skills

A. Prosthesis

B. Activities of daily living (ADL)

C. Restorative nursing care

D. Disability

E. Atrophy

F. Restorative aide

G. Rehabilitation

Fill in the Blanks

8. What is the function of the nervous system?

_____

_____

9. The central nervous system consists of

_____.

10. The peripheral nervous system involves

_____.

11. The cerebral cortex controls _____

_____

_____

_____.

12. The _____ controls balance and the smooth movements of voluntary muscles.

13. The spinal cord lies within the _____

_____.

14. What is the function of cerebral spinal fluid?

_____

_____

15. _____ nerves conduct impulses between the brain and the head, neck, chest, and abdomen.

16. A stroke is _____

_____

_____.

17. Brain damage occurs with a stroke. The functions lost depend on _____

_____.

18. Symptoms of multiple sclerosis usually occur between the ages of _____.

19. Head injuries can involve the _____, _____, and

_____.

20. List four common causes of spinal cord injuries.

A. _____

B. _____

C. _____

D. _____

21. Quadriplegia is _____

_____.

22. A spinal cord injury at the _____ level causes loss of muscle function below the chest.

23. A disability occurring before 22 years of age is called

_____.

24. Mental retardation involves _____

_____

_____.

25. Which developmental disability does an extra 21st chromosome cause?

_____

26. Define the following terms:

A. Abduction

_____

_____

B. Extension

_____

_____

C. Dorsiflexion

_____

_____

D. External rotation

_____

_____

E. Supination

_____

_____

27. The focus of rehabilitation is on

_____.

When improvement is not possible, the goal is to

_____.

28. Rehabilitation and restorative nursing programs do the following:

A. _____

B. _____

29. The person with a disability needs to adjust

_____,

_____,

_____,

and _____.

30. When does the rehabilitation process start?

_____

_____

31. Aphasia means _____

_____.

32. Doctors order bedrest to:

A. _____

B. _____

C. _____

D. _____

33. Define the following types of bedrest.

A. Bedrest

_____

_____

B. Strict bedrest

_____

_____

34. Common sites for contractures are the

_____,

_____,

_____,

_____,

_____,

_____,

and _____.

35. Describe two purposes of footboards.

A. _____

_____

B. _____

_____

36. _____ keep elbows, wrists, thumbs, fingers, ankles, and knees in normal position.

37. Define the following terms:

A. Active range-of-motion exercises

_____

_____

B. Passive range-of-motion exercises

_____

_____

C. Active-assistive range-of-motion exercises

_____

_____

38. You have performed active-assistive range-of-motion exercise on Ms. Merlin's right knee. What do you need to report and record?

A. _____

B. _____

C. _____

D. _____

E. _____

39. Which range-of-motion exercises are done to the knee?

A. _____

B. _____

40. What information do you need from the nurse and the care plan before you assist a person with ambulation?

A. _____

B. _____

C. _____

D. _____

E. _____

41. You are assisting Mr. Lang to ambulate. He begins to fall. What should you do?

_____

_____

42. A cane is held on the _____

side of the body.

43. Explain how to use a walker correctly.

_____

_____

_____

_____

_____

_____

44. Braces are used to:

A. _____

B. _____

C. _____

45. Ms. Norris wears a brace on her right ankle. How will you know when you need to apply and remove the brace?

_____

46. Successful rehabilitation depends on the person's

_____.

47. All members of the health team help the person

regain _____

and _____.

48. Every part of your job focuses on _____

_____.

49. To promote the person's quality of life, you need to:

A. _____

B. _____

C. _____

D. _____

E. _____

F. _____

G. _____

50. Mr. Romero is making slow progress in therapy. You hear a therapist shout at him. What should you do?

_____

_____

Circle the BEST Answer

51. Which statement about disabilities is *false?*
    A. Often more than one function is lost.
    B. The person may depend totally or in part on others for basic needs.
    C. The degree of disability affects how much function is possible.
    D. All disabilities are permanent.

52. The largest part of the brain is the
    A. Medulla
    B. Cerebrum
    C. Pons
    D. Hemisphere

53. Which is *not* an age-related change in the nervous system?
    A. Nerve cells are lost.
    B. Nerve conduction and reflexes speed up.
    C. Blood flow to the brain is reduced.
    D. Brain cells are lost over time.

54. This nervous system disorder is a slow, progressive disorder with no cure. Degeneration of a part of brain occurs.
    A. Head injury
    B. Multiple sclerosis
    C. Parkinson's disease
    D. Mental retardation

55. All head injuries are serious.
    A. True
    B. False

56. This term is applied to a group of disorders involving muscle weakness or poor muscle control.
    A. Developmental disability
    B. Cerebral palsy
    C. Down syndrome
    D. Mental retardation

57. This term means bending a body part.
    A. Adduction
    B. Rotation
    C. Flexion
    D. Pronation

58. Bending the foot down at the ankle is called
    A. Hyperextension
    B. Internal rotation
    C. Plantar flexion
    D. Rotation

59. When performing range-of-motion exercises, you must do all of the following *except*
    A. Exercise only the joints the nurse tells you to.
    B. Expose only the body part being exercised.
    C. Support the part being exercised.
    D. Move the joint with quick, firm movements.

60. In some centers only physical or occupational therapists do neck exercises.
    A. True
    B. False

61. Rehabilitation starts with
    A. Exercises
    B. Bladder training
    C. Preventing complications
    D. Self-care activities

62. Inactivity affects every body system.
    A. True
    B. False

63. Which measure will *not* help prevent the complications of bedrest?
    A. Good alignment
    B. Range-of-motion exercises
    C. Frequent position changes
    D. Doing as much for the person as possible

64. You promote a person's rehabilitation by
    A. Rushing the person
    B. Applying assistive (self-help) devices as ordered
    C. Feeling sorry for the person
    D. Focusing on what the person cannot do

65. Which device prevents external rotation of the hips and legs?
    A. A trochanter roll
    B. A hip abduction wedge
    C. A bed cradle
    D. A footboard

66. You need to help Mr. Lange with ambulation. He is unsteady. Which is *incorrect?*
    A. Apply a gait belt over his clothing.
    B. Help him to stand by grasping the gait belt at each side.
    C. Encourage him to stand erect with his head up and his back straight.
    D. Encourage him to walk slowly and to slide his feet.

67. Ms. Mann is learning to walk with crutches. Which will *not* promote her safety?
    A. Wearing flat street shoes with nonskid soles
    B. Wearing loose clothes and long skirts
    C. Replacing worn or torn crutch tips
    D. Keeping the crutches within her reach

68. Families are often a valuable part of the rehabilitation team.
    A. True
    B. False

69. Which is *not* a nursing assistant responsibility in rehabilitation?
    A. Knowing and following the person's care plan
    B. Preventing pressure ulcers
    C. Discussing the person's progress with the family
    D. Performing range-of-motion exercises as directed

70. Rehabilitation and restorative care is
    A. A team effort
    B. The doctor's responsibility
    C. Provided by physical and occupational therapists
    D. Not a focus of nursing centers

71. Family members are discouraged from participating in the person's rehabilitation.
    A. True
    B. False

Additional Learning Activities

1. Do you have a family member or a friend with a physical disability? Interview the person if he or she is willing.
   A. Discuss how the disability affects ADL.
   B. Is the person involved in rehabilitation?
   C. Are community programs available when needed?
   D. Does the person use self-help devices?
   E. Have any changes been made in the person's home to help maintain independence?
   F. Has the person's job been affected by the disability?

2. Read the vignette; then answer the questions that follow.

   Ms. Barbara Brown is 60 years old. She is a widow. She works as a secretary for a lawyer. Ms. Brown had a stroke. Her right side is paralyzed. She has facial drooping. Her speech is affected. She has trouble expressing herself. She needs assistance with all ADL. She is receiving rehabilitation in a skilled nursing center. Her goal is to learn to walk and to care for herself, so she can go home. She is afraid she will never be able to work as a secretary again.

   Ms. Brown is motivated and works hard with the rehabilitation team. She tells you that she is embarrassed by her appearance. She wants to eat in her room as she feels she is messy. She told the nurse that she does not want visitors until she is doing better.

A. How does Ms. Brown's stroke affect her physically, psychologically, socially, and economically?

(1) Privacy

(2) Personal choice

(3) Be free from abuse and mistreatment

B. What effect does the stroke have on Ms. Brown's
self-esteem?

C. What health team members might be involved in
Ms. Brown's rehabilitation?

E. What measures will promote her safety?

D. How can the health team promote Ms. Brown's
right to:

20 Restraint Alternatives and Safe Restraint Use

OBJECTIVES

The questions and student activities in this chapter will help you meet these objectives.
- Define the key terms listed in Chapter 20
- Describe the purpose and complications of restraints
- Identify restraint alternatives
- Explain how to use restraints safely
- Perform the procedure described in Chapter 20

Study Questions

Matching

Match each term with the correct definition.

1. _____ Any action that punishes or penalizes a person

2. _____ A restraint attached to the person's body and to a fixed (non-movable) object

3. _____ Any item, object, device, garment, material, or drug that limits or restricts a person's freedom of movement or access to one's body

4. _____ A restraint near but not directly attached to the person's body

A. Restraint

B. Passive physical restraint

C. Active physical restraint

D. Discipline

Fill in the Blanks

5. _____,

_____,

and _____

have guidelines about restraint use. So do

_____ and

_____.

6. List seven risks of restraint use.

A. _____

B. _____

C. _____

D. _____

E. _____

F. _____

G. _____

7. Restraints cannot be used for staff convenience. Convenience is any action that:

    A. _____

    B. _____

    C. _____

8. The nurse retrains Mr. Gomez to the chair in his room so she can make rounds without being interrupted.

    This action is _____.

9. Restraints are used only when necessary to

    _____

    _____.

10. According to the Omnibus Budget Reconciliation Act of 1987 (OBRA) and Centers for Medicare & Medicaid Assistance (CMS), physical restraints include these points:

    A. _____

    _____

    B. _____

    C. _____

    D. _____

11. Drugs are restraints if they:

    A. _____

    B. _____

12. The doctor may order drugs to help persons who are confused or agitated. What is the goal?

    _____

    _____

13. You must follow safety measures whenever restraints are used. You must also remember the following:

    A. _____

    _____

    B. _____

    _____

    C. _____

    _____

    D. _____

    _____

    E. _____

    _____

    F. _____

    _____

    G. _____

    _____

    H. _____

    _____

    I. _____

    _____

    J. _____

    _____

    K. _____

    _____

    L. _____

    _____

    M. _____

    _____

14. Mrs. Monroe's doctor writes an order for a restraint. What must the doctor's order include?

    A. _____

    B. _____

    C. _____

    D. _____

15. The nurse tells you to apply a wrist restraint to Mr. Clark's right wrist. You do not understand why the restraint is being used. What should you do and why?

    _____

    _____

16. You are applying a belt restraint to Mr. Norris. He is confused and resists your efforts. What should you do?

    _____

    _____

17. Before you apply any restraint, what information do you need from the nurse and the care plan?

    A. _____

    _____

    B. _____

    _____

    C. _____

    _____

    D. _____

    _____

    E. _____

    _____

    F. _____

    _____

    G. _____

    _____

H. _____

    _____

I. _____

    _____

J. _____

    _____

K. _____

    _____

18. You apply a belt restraint to Ms. Monroe when she is in her wheelchair. What information must you report to the nurse?

    A. _____

    B. _____

    C. _____

    D. _____

    E. _____

    F. _____

    G. _____

    H. _____

    I. _____

    J. _____

19. Mr. Clark has a wrist restraint on his right wrist. You are checking the circulation in his right wrist. What signs and symptoms must you report to the nurse at once?

    A. _____

    B. _____

    C. _____

    D. _____

20. Why are persons restrained in the supine position monitored constantly?

_____

_____

21. What is the purpose of bed rail covers and gap protectors?

_____

_____

22. When applying a restraint to a person's chest, you must

_____

_____

_____.

23. Criss-crossing vest restraints in back can cause

_____.

24. You must remove Mr. Clark's restraint at least every 2 hours. What care measures do you need to perform before you reapply the restraint?

A. _____

B. _____

C. _____

D. _____

Circle the BEST Answer

25. Physical restraints
    A. Restrict freedom of movement or access to one's body
    B. Must be used to control a person's behavior
    C. Are effective in preventing falls
    D. Should never be used

26. Which of the following is a physical restraint?
    A. The person is moved closer to the nurses' station.
    B. The person is taken to a supervised activity.
    C. The person wears padded hip protectors under his or her clothing.
    D. The person's chair is placed so close to the wall that the person cannot move.

27. The most serious risk from restraints is
    A. Loss of dignity
    B. Fractured hip
    C. Increased agitation
    D. Death from strangulation

28. Which is *not* a restraint alternative?
    A. An exercise program is provided.
    B. A floor cushion is placed next to the person's bed.
    C. The person's bed sheets are tucked in so tightly that the person cannot move.
    D. Extra time is spent with the person who is restless.

29. Restraints cannot be used without consent.
    A. True
    B. False

30. Mr. Norris is confused. He cannot give informed consent for restraint use. Who does so for him?
    A. The doctor
    B. The RN
    C. The center's administrator
    D. Mr. Norris's legal representative

31. You may need to apply restraints or care for persons who are restrained. Which action is unsafe?
    A. Using the restraint noted in the person's care plan
    B. Using only restraints that have manufacturer instructions and warning labels
    C. Using a restraint to position a person on the toilet
    D. Padding bony areas and skin

32. For safe use of restraints
    A. Keep bed rails down when using vest, jacket, or belt restraints.
    B. Position the person in the supine position when using vest, belt, or jacket restraints.
    C. Tie restraints according to center policy.
    D. Secure restraints to the bed rail.

33. Back cushions are used when a person is restrained in a chair.
    A. True
    B. False

34. How often do you need to check the person's circulation if mitt, wrist, or ankle restraints are used?
    A. At least every 15 minutes
    B. At least every 30 minutes
    C. Every hour
    D. Every 2 hours

35. Which restraints limit arm movements?
    A. Mitt restraints
    B. Wrist restraints
    C. Belt restraints
    D. Vest restraints

36. Which type of restraint is the *most* restrictive?
    A. A mitt restraint
    B. A wrist restraint
    C. A belt restraint
    D. A vest restraint

37. You are applying a wrist restraint. The person is in bed. Where should you tie the straps?
    A. To the headboard
    B. To the bed rail out of the person's reach
    C. To the footboard
    D. To the moveable part of the bed frame out of the person's reach

Additional Learning Activities

1. Read the vignette; then answer the questions that follow.

   Ms. Ann Bert is a resident of Valley View Nursing Center. She has pneumonia. She is receiving oxygen by nasal cannula and has an IV in her left arm. Ms. Bert is very restless. She tries to get out of bed. She pulled her IV catheter out this morning. She also takes her nasal cannula off frequently. She keeps calling for her daughter and shouting, "I need to go home."

   A. What are Ms. Bert's safety needs?

   B. What might be some of the causes for Ms. Bert's behaviors?

   C. What restraint alternatives might be tried?

2. You are caring for a person who is restrained. List some things you can do to protect the person's quality of life. Discuss how you would want to be treated.

3. Under the supervision of your instructor, practice the procedures for applying restraints with a classmate.
   A. Use the procedure checklist on pages 238 -240 to evaluate your technique. Remember that restraints can cause serious injury and even death. They must always be applied correctly.

4. Under the supervision of your instructor, allow a classmate to practice applying restraints to you. Discuss how it feels to be restrained. Answer these questions.
   A. Did you feel safe? Explain.

   B. Did you feel comfortable? Explain.

   C. Did you feel in control? Explain.

   D. What fears did you have?

5. Imagine that you are in a nursing center. You are having a lot pain. You do not know the staff. The medication you are taking makes you drowsy. You are not sure what day it is. You have an IV in your right arm and a tube in your nose. You are frightened.
   A. What behaviors might you have?

B. What could be some reasons for your behavior?

D. Would you feel safer and less fearful if you were restrained?

C. Might the staff believe that you are confused? Explain.

E. What measures would make you feel safe and less fearful?

Procedure Checklists

Hand Washing

Name: _____   Date: _____

Procedure	S	U	Comments
1. Reviewed Safety Alert.	____	____	_____
2. Made sure to have soap, paper towels, orange stick or nail file, and a wastebasket. Collected missing items.	____	____	_____
3. Pushed watch up 4 to 5 inches. Also pushed up uniform sleeves.	____	____	_____
4. Stood away from the sink so that clothes did not touch the sink. Stood so the soap and faucet were easy to reach.	____	____	_____
5. Turned on and adjusted the water until it felt warm.	____	____	_____
6. Wet wrists and hands. Kept hands lower than elbows.	____	____	_____
7. Applied about 1 teaspoon of soap to hands.	____	____	_____
8. Rubbed palms together and interlaced fingers to work up a good lather for at least 15 seconds.	____	____	_____
9. Washed each hand and wrist thoroughly. Cleaned well between the fingers.	____	____	_____
10. Cleaned under the fingernails. Rubbed the finger tips against the palms.	____	____	_____
11. Cleaned under fingernails with a nail file or orange stick.	____	____	_____
12. Rinsed wrists and hands well. Water flowed from the arms to the hands.	____	____	_____
13. Repeated steps 7 through 12, if needed.	____	____	_____
14. Dried wrists and hands with paper towels. Patted dry starting at the fingertips.	____	____	_____
15. Discarded the paper towels.	____	____	_____
16. Turned off faucets with clean paper towels. Used a clean paper towel for each faucet.	____	____	_____
17. Discarded paper towels.	____	____	_____

Date of Satisfactory Completion _____   Instructor's Initials _____

Removing Gloves

Name: _____   Date: _____

Procedure	S	U	Comments
1. Reviewed Safety Alert.	_____	_____	_____
2. Made sure that glove only touched glove.	_____	_____	_____
3. Grasped a glove just below the cuff. Grasped it on the outside.	_____	_____	_____
4. Pulled the glove down over the hand so it was inside out.	_____	_____	_____
5. Held the removed glove with the other gloved hand.	_____	_____	_____
6. Reached inside the other glove. Used the first two fingers of the ungloved hand.	_____	_____	_____
7. Pulled the glove down (inside out) over the hand and the other glove.	_____	_____	_____
8. Discarded the gloves. Followed center policy.	_____	_____	_____
9. Decontaminated hands.	_____	_____	_____

Date of Satisfactory Completion _____ Instructor's Initials _____

Wearing a Mask

Name: _____   Date: _____

Procedure	**S**	**U**	**Comments**
1. Practiced hand hygiene.	____	____	_____
2. Picked up the mask by its upper ties. Did not touch the part that would cover the face.	____	____	_____
3. Placed the mask over the nose and mouth.	____	____	_____
4. Placed the upper strings above the ears. Tied them at the back of the head.	____	____	_____
5. Tied the lower strings at the back of the neck. The lower part of the mask was under the chin.	____	____	_____
6. Pinched the metal band around the nose. The top of the mask was snug over the nose. If glasses were worn, the mask was snug under the bottom of the glasses.	____	____	_____
7. Decontaminated hands. Put on gloves.	____	____	_____
8. Provided care. Avoided coughing, sneezing, and unnecessary talking.	____	____	_____
9. Changed the mask if it became moist or contaminated.	____	____	_____
10. Removed the mask as follows:			
a. Removed the gloves.	____	____	_____
b. Decontaminated hands.	____	____	_____
c. Untied the lower strings.	____	____	_____
d. Untied the top strings.	____	____	_____
e. Held the top strings. Removed the mask.	____	____	_____
f. Brought the strings together. The inside of the mask folded together. Did not touch the inside of the mask.	____	____	_____
11. Discarded the mask. Followed center policy.	____	____	_____
12. Decontaminated hands.	____	____	_____

Date of Satisfactory Completion _____   Instructor's Initials _____

Donning and Removing a Gown

Name: _____   Date: _____

Procedure	S	U	Comments
1. Removed the watch and all jewelry.	____	____	_____
2. Rolled up uniform sleeves.	____	____	_____
3. Practiced hand hygiene.	____	____	_____
4. Put on a face mask and eyewear, if required. (Followed procedure for wearing a mask.)	____	____	_____
5. Held a clean gown out in front of you. Let it unfold. Did not shake the gown.	____	____	_____
6. Put the hands and arms through the sleeves.	____	____	_____
7. Made sure the gown covered the front of the uniform. It was snug at the neck.	____	____	_____
8. Tied the strings at the back of the neck.	____	____	_____
9. Overlapped the back of the gown. Made sure it covered the uniform. The gown was snug, not loose.	____	____	_____
10. Tied the waist strings at the back.	____	____	_____
11. Put on the gloves.	____	____	_____
12. Provided care.	____	____	_____
13. Removed and discarded the gloves. Decontaminated hands.	____	____	_____
14. Removed and discarded the mask following center policy.	____	____	_____
15. Removed the gown:			
a. Untied the waist strings.	____	____	_____
b. Decontaminated hands.	____	____	_____
c. Untied the neck strings. Did not touch the outside of the gown.	____	____	_____
d. Pulled the gown down from the shoulder.	____	____	_____
e. Turned the gown inside out as it was removed. Held it at the inside shoulder seams and brought your hands together.	____	____	_____
16. Rolled up the gown away from you. Kept it inside out.	____	____	_____
17. Discarded the gown. Followed center policy.	____	____	_____
18. Removed and discarded eyewear following center policy.	____	____	_____
19. Decontaminated hands.	____	____	_____
20. Opened the door using a paper towel. Discarded it as you left.	____	____	_____

Date of Satisfactory Completion _____   Instructor's Initials _____

Helping the Falling Person

Name: _____   Date: _____

Procedure	S	U	Comments
1. Stood with your feet apart. Kept your back straight.	_____	_____	_____
2. Brought the person close to your body as fast as possible. Used the gait belt, or wrapped your arms around the person's waist. The person could also be held under the arms.	_____	_____	_____
3. Moved your leg so the person's buttocks rested on it. Moved the leg near the person.	_____	_____	_____
4. Lowered the person to the floor. The person slid down your leg to the floor. Bent at the hips and knees as the person was lowered.	_____	_____	_____
5. Called a nurse to check the person. Stayed with the person.	_____	_____	_____
6. Helped the nurse return the person to bed. Got other staff to help if needed.	_____	_____	_____
7. Reported the following to the nurse:			
• How the fall occurred	_____	_____	_____
• How far the person walked	_____	_____	_____
• How activity was tolerated before the fall	_____	_____	_____
• Complaints before the fall	_____	_____	_____
• How much help the person needed while walking	_____	_____	_____
8. Completed an incident report.	_____	_____	_____

Date of Satisfactory Completion _____   Instructor's Initials _____

Applying Heat and Cold Applications

Name: _____   Date: _____

Quality of Life	S	U	Comments
• Knocked before entering the person's room	____	____	_____
• Addressed the person by name	____	____	_____
• Introduced yourself by name and title	____	____	_____

Pre-Procedure

1. Followed Delegation Guidelines. Reviewed Safety Alert.
2. Explained the procedure to the person.
3. Practiced hand hygiene.
4. Collected needed equipment.
5. Identified the person. Checked the ID bracelet against the assignment sheet. Called the person by name.
6. Provided for privacy.

Procedure

7. Prepared the application. Followed center procedures and the manufacturer's instructions
8. Placed a dry application in a cover.
9. Placed the application on the affected part. Noted the time.
10. Secured the application in place with ties, tape, or rolled gauze. Did not use pins.
11. Unscreened the person. Placed the signal light within reach.
12. Raised or lowered bed rails. Followed the care plan.
13. Checked the area every 5 minutes. Checked for signs and symptoms of complications. Removed the application if any occurred. Told the nurse at once.
14. Removed the application at the specified time. (If the bed rail was up, lowered it for this step.)

Post-Procedure

15. Provided for comfort.
16. Unscreened the person.
17. Placed the signal light within reach.
18. Raised or lowered bed rails. Followed the care plan.
19. Completed a safety check of the room.
20. Cleaned the sitz with disinfectant solution. Wore utility gloves.
21. Cleaned and returned reusable items to their proper place. Followed center policy for soiled linen. Wore gloves for this step.
22. Discarded the gloves. Decontaminated hands.
23. Reported and recorded observations.

Date of Satisfactory Completion _____   Instructor's Initials _____

Using a Fire Extinguisher

Name: _____   Date: _____

Procedure	S	U	Comments
1. Pulled the fire alarm.	_____	_____	_____
2. Got the nearest fire extinguisher.	_____	_____	_____
3. Carried it upright.	_____	_____	_____
4. Took it to the fire.	_____	_____	_____
5. Removed the safety pin.	_____	_____	_____
6. Directed the hose at the base of the fire.	_____	_____	_____
7. Pushed the top handle down.	_____	_____	_____
8. Swept the hose slowly back and forth at the base of the fire.	_____	_____	_____

Date of Satisfactory Completion _____   Instructor's Initials _____

Adult CPR—One Rescuer

Name: _____   Date: _____

Procedure	S	U	Comments
1. Checked if the person was responding. Tapped or gently shook the person, called the person by name and shouted "Are you OK?"	_____	_____	_____
2. Called for help.	_____	_____	_____
3. Positioned the person supine. Logrolled the person so there was no twisting of the spine. Placed the person's arms alongside the body.	_____	_____	_____
4. Opened the airway. Used the head-tilt/chin-lift method.	_____	_____	_____
5. Checked for breathing. Looked to see if the chest rose and fell. Listened for the escape of air. Felt for the flow of air on your cheek.	_____	_____	_____
6. Gave 2 slow breaths if the person was not breathing or was not breathing adequately. Each breath took 2 seconds. Let the person's lungs deflate between breaths.			
7. Checked for a carotid pulse and for breathing, coughing, and moving. This took 5 to 10 seconds. Used one hand to keep the airway open with the head-tilt/chin-lift method. Started chest compressions if there was no sign of circulation.	_____	_____	_____
8. Gave 100 chest compressions per minute. Gave 15 compressions and then 2 slow breaths.	_____	_____	_____
a. Established a rhythm and counted out loud. (Try: "1 and, 2 and, 3 and, 4 and, 5 and, 6 and, 7 and, 8 and, 9 and, 10 and, 11 and, 12 and, 13 and, 14 and, 15.")	_____	_____	_____
b. Opened the airway, and gave 2 slow breaths.	_____	_____	_____
c. Repeated this step until 4 cycles of 15 compressions and 2 breaths were given.	_____	_____	_____
9. Checked for a carotid pulse. Also checked for breathing, coughing, and moving.	_____	_____	_____
10. Continued with 15 compressions and 2 slow breaths if the person had no signs of circulation. Started with chest compressions. Checked for circulation every few minutes.	_____	_____	_____
11. Did the following if the person had signs of circulation:			
a. Checked for breathing.	_____	_____	_____
b. Positioned the person in the recovery position if the person was breathing.	_____	_____	_____
c. Monitored breathing and circulation.	_____	_____	_____
12. Did the following if the person had signs of circulation but breathing was absent:			
a. Gave 1 rescue breath every 5 seconds (10 to 12 breaths per minute).	_____	_____	_____
b. Monitored circulation.	_____	_____	_____

Date of Satisfactory Completion _____   Instructor's Initials _____

Adult CPR—Two Rescuers

Name: _____   Date: _____

Procedure	S	U	Comments

Procedure   **S**   **U**   **Comments**

1. Checked if the person was responding. Tapped or gently shook the person, called the person by name, and shouted "Are you OK?" One rescuer called for help.   _____ _____ _____

2. Opened the airway and checked for breathing. Used the head-tilt/chin-lift method.   _____ _____ _____

3. Gave 2 slow rescue breaths if the person was not breathing or if breathing was inadequate. Let the lungs deflate between breaths.   _____ _____ _____

4. Checked for a pulse using the carotid artery. Checked for breathing, coughing, and moving.   _____ _____ _____

5. Performed 2-person CPR if there were no signs of circulation.   _____ _____ _____

    a. One rescuer gave 100 chest compressions per minute. Counted out loud in a rhythm. ("1 and, 2 and, 3 and, 4 and, 5 and, 6 and, 7 and, 8 and, 9 and, 10 and, 11 and, 12 and, 13 and, 14 and, 15.")   _____ _____ _____

    b. The other rescuer gave 2 slow breaths after every 15 compressions. Paused for the breaths. Continued chest compressions after the breaths.   _____ _____ _____

6. One rescuer did the following after 4 cycles of 15 compressions and 2 breaths:

    a. Gave 2 slow breaths.   _____ _____ _____

    b. Checked for circulation—carotid pulse, breathing, coughing, and moving.   _____ _____ _____

7. Continued with 15 compressions and 2 slow breaths if the person had no signs of circulation. Started with chest compressions.   _____ _____ _____

Date of Satisfactory Completion _____   Instructor's Initials _____

FBAO—The Responsive Adult

Name: _____   Date: _____

Procedure	**S**	**U**	**Comments**
1. Asked the person if he or she was choking.	____	____	_____
2. Asked if the person could cough or speak.	____	____	_____
3. Gave abdominal thrusts.			
a. Stood behind the person.	____	____	_____
b. Wrapped your arms around the person's waist.	____	____	_____
c. Made a fist with one hand.	____	____	_____
d. Placed the thumb side of the fist against the abdomen. The fist was in the middle above the navel and below the end of the sternum (breastbone).	____	____	_____
e. Grasped the fist with the other hand.	____	____	_____
f. Pressed the fist and hand into the person's abdomen with a quick, upward thrust.	____	____	_____
g. Repeated thrusts until the object was expelled or the person lost consciousness.	____	____	_____
4. Lowered the unresponsive person to the floor or ground. Positioned the person supine.	____	____	_____
5. Called for help.	____	____	_____
6. Did a finger sweep to check for a foreign object.	____	____	_____
a. Opened the person's mouth. Used the tongue-jaw lift method.	____	____	_____
(1) Grasped the person's tongue and lower jaw with the thumb and fingers.	____	____	_____
(2) Lifted the lower jaw upward.	____	____	_____
b. Inserted the other index finger into the mouth along the side of the cheek and deep into the throat. The finger was at the base of the tongue.	____	____	_____
c. Formed a hook with the index finger.	____	____	_____
d. Tried to dislodge and remove the object. Did not push it deeper into the throat.	____	____	_____
e. Grasped and removed the object if it was within reach.	____	____	_____
7. Opened the airway with the head-tilt/chin-lift method.	____	____	_____
8. Gave 1 or 2 rescue breaths.	____	____	_____
9. Repositioned the person's head if the chest did not rise. Gave 1 or 2 rescue breaths.	____	____	_____
10. Gave up to 5 abdominal thrusts.	____	____	_____
11. Repeated steps 6 through 10 (finger sweeps, rescue breathing, and abdominal thrusts) until rescue breathing was effective. Started CPR if necessary.	____	____	_____

Date of Satisfactory Completion _____   Instructor's Initials _____

FBAO—The Unresponsive Adult

Name: _____   Date: _____

Procedure	S	U	Comments
1. Checked to see if the person was responding.	_____	_____	_____
2. Called for help.	_____	_____	_____
3. Logrolled the person to the supine position with his or her face up. Arms were at the sides.	_____	_____	_____
4. Opened the airway. Used the head-tilt/chin-lift method.	_____	_____	_____
5. Checked for breathing.	_____	_____	_____
6. Gave 1 or 2 slow rescue breaths. Repositioned the person's head and opened the airway if the chest did not rise. Gave 1 or 2 rescue breaths.	_____	_____	_____
7. Gave 5 abdominal thrusts if the person could not be ventilated.	_____	_____	_____
a. Straddled the person's thighs.	_____	_____	_____
b. Placed the heel of one hand against the abdomen. It was in the middle above the navel and below the end of the sternum (breastbone).	_____	_____	_____
c. Placed the second hand on top of the first hand.	_____	_____	_____
d. Pressed both hands into the abdomen with a quick, upward thrust. Gave 5 thrusts.	_____	_____	_____
8. Did a finger sweep to check for a foreign object.	_____	_____	_____
9. Repeated steps 6 through 8 until rescue breathing was effective. Started CPR if necessary.	_____	_____	_____

Date of Satisfactory Completion _____ Instructor's Initials _____

Taking a Temperature With a Glass Thermometer

Name: _____   Date: _____

Quality of Life	S	U	Comments
• Knocked before entering the person's room	____	____	_____
• Addressed the person by name	____	____	_____
• Introduced yourself by name and title	____	____	_____

Pre-Procedure

1. Followed Delegation Guidelines. Reviewed Safety Alerts. ____ ____ _____
2. Explained the procedure to the person. ____ ____ _____
3. Collected the following:
   - • Oral or rectal thermometer and holder ____ ____ _____
   - • Tissues ____ ____ _____
   - • Plastic covers if used ____ ____ _____
   - • Gloves ____ ____ _____
   - • Toilet tissue (rectal temperature) ____ ____ _____
   - • Water-soluble lubricant (rectal temperature) ____ ____ _____
   - • Towel (axillary temperature) ____ ____ _____
4. Practiced hand hygiene. ____ ____ _____
5. Identified the person. Checked the ID bracelet against the assignment sheet. Called the person by name. ____ ____ _____
6. Provided for privacy. ____ ____ _____

Procedure

7. Put on the gloves. ____ ____ _____
8. Rinsed the thermometer in cold water if it was soaking in a disinfectant. Dried it with tissues. ____ ____ _____
9. Checked for breaks, cracks, or chips. ____ ____ _____
10. Shook down the thermometer below the lowest number. ____ ____ _____
11. Inserted it into a plastic cover, if used. ____ ____ _____
12. For an oral temperature:
    a. Asked the person to moisten the lips. ____ ____ _____
    b. Placed the bulb end of the thermometer under the tongue. ____ ____ _____
    c. Asked the person to close the lips around the thermometer to hold it in place. ____ ____ _____
    d. Asked the person not to talk. Reminded the person not to bite down on the thermometer. ____ ____ _____
    e. Left it in place for 2 to 3 minutes or as required by center policy. ____ ____ _____
13. For a rectal temperature:
    a. Positioned the person in Sims' position. ____ ____ _____
    b. Put a small amount of lubricant on a tissue. Lubricated the bulb end of the thermometer. ____ ____ _____
    c. Folded back top linens to expose the anal area. ____ ____ _____

Continued

Procedure—cont'd   S   U   Comments

d. Raised the upper buttock to expose the anus. _____ _____ _____

e. Inserted the thermometer 1 inch into the rectum. Did not _____ _____ _____
   force the thermometer.

f. Held the thermometer in place for 2 minutes or as required by _____ _____ _____
   center policy. Did not let go of it while it was in the rectum.

14. For an axillary temperature:

a. Helped the person remove an arm from the gown. Did not _____ _____ _____
   expose the person.

b. Dried the axilla with the towel. _____ _____ _____

c. Placed the bulb end of the thermometer in the center of the _____ _____ _____
   axilla.

d. Asked the person to place the arm over the chest to hold the _____ _____ _____
   thermometer in place. Held it and the arm in place if he or
   she could not help.

e. Left the thermometer in place for 5 to 10 minutes or as _____ _____ _____
   required by center policy.

15. Removed the thermometer. _____ _____ _____

16. Used tissues to remove the plastic cover. Wiped the thermo- _____ _____ _____
    meter with a tissue if no cover was used. Wiped from the stem
    to the bulb end.

17. For a rectal temperature:

a. Placed used toilet tissue on several thicknesses of clean _____ _____ _____
   toilet tissue.

b. Placed the thermometer on clean toilet tissue. _____ _____ _____

c. Wiped the anal area to remove excess lubricant and any feces. _____ _____ _____

d. Covered the person. _____ _____ _____

18. For an axillary temperature: Helped the person put the gown _____ _____ _____
    back on.

19. Read the thermometer. _____ _____ _____

20. Recorded the person's name and temperature on the note pad or _____ _____ _____
    assignment sheet. Wrote R for a rectal temperature. Wrote A for
    an axillary temperature.

21. Shook down the thermometer. _____ _____ _____

22. Cleaned it according to center policy. _____ _____ _____

23. Discarded tissue and disposed of toilet tissue. _____ _____ _____

24. Removed the gloves. Decontaminated hands. _____ _____ _____

Post-Procedure

25. Provided for comfort. _____ _____ _____

26. Placed the signal light within reach. _____ _____ _____

27. Unscreened the person. _____ _____ _____

28. Completed a safety check of the room. _____ _____ _____

29. Decontaminated hands. _____ _____ _____

30. Reported any abnormal temperature to the nurse. Recorded the _____ _____ _____
    temperature in the proper place. Noted the temperature site.

Date of Satisfactory Completion _____ Instructor's Initials _____

Taking a Temperature With an Electronic Thermometer

Name: _____   Date: _____

Quality of Life	S	U	Comments
• Knocked before entering the person's room	____	____	_____
• Addressed the person by name	____	____	_____
• Introduced yourself by name and title	____	____	_____

Pre-Procedure

1. Followed Delegation Guidelines. Reviewed Safety Alert.   ____ ____ _____
2. Explained the procedure to the person. For an oral temperature,   ____ ____ _____
   asked the person not to eat, drink, smoke, or chew gum for at
   least 15 to 20 minutes.
3. Collected the following:
   • Thermometer—electronic or tympanic membrane   ____ ____ _____
   • Probe (Blue for an oral or axillary temperature. Red for a   ____ ____ _____
     rectal temperature.)
   • Probe covers   ____ ____ _____
   • Toilet tissue (rectal temperature)   ____ ____ _____
   • Water-soluble lubricant (rectal temperature)   ____ ____ _____
   • Gloves   ____ ____ _____
   • Towel (axillary temperature)   ____ ____ _____
4. Plugged the probe into the thermometer. (This is not done for a   ____ ____ _____
   tympanic membrane thermometer.)
5. Practiced hand hygiene.   ____ ____ _____
6. Identified the person. Checked the ID bracelet against the as-   ____ ____ _____
   signment sheet. Called the person by name.

Procedure

7. Provided for privacy.   ____ ____ _____
8. Positioned the person for an oral, rectal, axillary, or tympanic   ____ ____ _____
   membrane temperature.
9. Put on gloves if contact with blood, body fluids, secretions, or   ____ ____ _____
   excretions was likely.
10. Inserted the probe into a probe cover.   ____ ____ _____
11. For an oral temperature:
    a. Asked the person to open the mouth and raise the tongue.   ____ ____ _____
    b. Placed the covered probe at the base of the tongue.   ____ ____ _____
    c. Asked the person to lower the tongue and close the mouth.   ____ ____ _____
12. For a rectal temperature:
    a. Placed some lubricant on toilet tissue.   ____ ____ _____
    b. Lubricated the end of the covered probe.   ____ ____ _____
    c. Exposed the anal area.   ____ ____ _____
    d. Raised the upper buttock.   ____ ____ _____

Continued

Procedure—cont'd   S   U   **Comments**

    e. Inserted the probe $\frac{1}{2}$ inch into the rectum.   _____ _____ _____

    f. Held the probe in place.   _____ _____ _____

13. For an axillary temperature:

    a. Helped the person remove an arm from the gown. Did not expose the person.   _____ _____ _____

    b. Dried the axilla with the towel.   _____ _____ _____

    c. Placed the covered probe in the center of the axilla.   _____ _____ _____

    d. Placed the person's arm over the chest.   _____ _____ _____

    e. Held the probe in place.   _____ _____ _____

14. For a tympanic membrane temperature:

    a. Asked the person to turn the head so the ear was in front of you.   _____ _____ _____

    b. Pulled up and back on the ear to straighten the ear canal.   _____ _____ _____

    c. Inserted the covered probe gently.   _____ _____ _____

15. Started the thermometer.   _____ _____ _____

16. Held the probe in place until a tone was heard or a flashing or steady light was seen.   _____ _____ _____

17. Read the temperature on the display.   _____ _____ _____

18. Removed the probe. Pressed the eject button to discard the cover.   _____ _____ _____

19. Recorded the person's name and temperature on the note pad or assignment sheet. Noted the temperature site.   _____ _____ _____

20. Returned the probe to the holder.   _____ _____ _____

21. Provided for comfort. Helped the person put the gown back on (axillary temperature). For a rectal temperature: _____ _____ _____

    a. Wiped the anal area with tissue to remove lubricant.   _____ _____ _____

    b. Covered the person.   _____ _____ _____

    c. Discarded used toilet tissue.   _____ _____ _____

    d. Removed the gloves. Decontaminated hands.   _____ _____ _____

Post-Procedure

22. Placed the signal light within reach.   _____ _____ _____

23. Unscreened the person.   _____ _____ _____

24. Completed a safety check of the room.   _____ _____ _____

25. Returned the thermometer to the charging unit.   _____ _____ _____

26. Decontaminated hands.   _____ _____ _____

27. Reported any abnormal temperature. Recorded the temperature in the proper place. Noted the temperature site.   _____ _____ _____

Date of Satisfactory Completion _____ Instructor's Initials _____

Taking a Radial Pulse

Name: _____   Date: _____

Quality of Life	S	U	Comments
• Knocked before entering the person's room	___	___	_____
• Addressed the person by name	___	___	_____
• Introduced yourself by name and title	___	___	_____

Pre-Procedure

1. Followed Delegation Guidelines. Reviewed Safety Alert. ___ ___ _____
2. Practiced hand hygiene. ___ ___ _____
3. Identified the person. Checked the ID bracelet against the assignment sheet. Called the person by name. ___ ___ _____
4. Explained the procedure to the person. ___ ___ _____
5. Provided for privacy. ___ ___ _____

Procedure

6. Had the person sit or lie down. ___ ___ _____
7. Located the radial pulse. Used your first 2 or 3 middle fingers. ___ ___ _____
8. Noted if the pulse was strong or weak, and regular or irregular. ___ ___ _____
9. Counted the pulse for 30 seconds. Multiplied the number of beats by 2. Or, counted the pulse for 1 minute as directed by the nurse or if required by center policy. ___ ___ _____
10. Counted the pulse for 1 minute if it was irregular. ___ ___ _____
11. Recorded the person's name and pulse on the note pad or assignment sheet. Noted the strength of the pulse. Noted if it was regular or irregular. ___ ___ _____

Post-Procedure

12. Provided for comfort. ___ ___ _____
13. Placed the signal light within reach. ___ ___ _____
14. Unscreened the person. ___ ___ _____
15. Completed a safety check of the room. ___ ___ _____
16. Decontaminated hands. ___ ___ _____
17. Reported and recorded the pulse rate and observations. ___ ___ _____

Date of Satisfactory Completion _____   Instructor's Initials _____

Taking an Apical Pulse

Name: _____   Date: _____

Quality of Life	S	U	Comments

- Knocked before entering the person's room
- Addressed the person by name
- Introduced yourself by name and title

Pre-Procedure

1. Followed Delegation Guidelines. Reviewed Safety Alert.
2. Collected a stethoscope and antiseptic wipes.
3. Practiced hand hygiene.
4. Identified the person. Checked the ID bracelet against the assignment sheet. Called the person by name.
5. Explained the procedure to the person.
6. Provided for privacy.

Procedure

7. Cleaned the earpieces and diaphragm with the wipes.
8. Had the person sit or lie down.
9. Exposed the nipple area of the left chest. Did not expose a woman's breasts.
10. Warmed the diaphragm in your palm.
11. Placed the earpieces in your ears.
12. Found the apical pulse. Placed the diaphragm 2 to 3 inches to the left of the breastbone and below the left nipple.
13. Counted the pulse for 1 minute. Noted if it was regular or irregular.
14. Covered the person. Removed the earpieces.
15. Recorded the person's name and pulse on the note pad or assignment sheet. Noted if the pulse was regular or irregular.

Post-Procedure

16. Provided for comfort.
17. Placed the signal light within reach.
18. Unscreened the person.
19. Completed a safety check of the room.
20. Cleaned the earpieces and diaphragm with the wipes.
21. Returned the stethoscope to its proper place.
22. Decontaminated hands.
23. Reported and recorded observations. Recorded the pulse rate with Ap for apical pulse.

Date of Satisfactory Completion _____   Instructor's Initials _____

Counting Respirations

Name: _____   Date: _____

Procedure	S	U	Comments
1. Followed Delegation Guidelines.	____	____	_____
2. Kept your fingers or the stethoscope over the pulse site.	____	____	_____
3. Did not tell the person that respirations were being counted.	____	____	_____
4. Began counting when the chest rose. Counted each rise and fall of the chest as 1 respiration.	____	____	_____
5. Noted the following:			
• If respirations were regular	____	____	_____
• If both sides of the chest rose equally	____	____	_____
• The depth of respirations	____	____	_____
• If the person had any pain or difficulty breathing	____	____	_____
6. Counted respirations for 30 seconds. Multiplied the number by 2. Counted for 1 minute, if required.	____	____	_____
7. Counted respirations for 1 minute if they were abnormal or irregular.	____	____	_____
8. Recorded the person's name, respiratory rate, and other observations on the note pad or assignment sheet.	____	____	_____

Post-Procedure

	S	U	Comments
9. Provided for comfort.	____	____	_____
10. Placed the signal light within reach.	____	____	_____
11. Completed a safety check of the room.	____	____	_____
12. Decontaminated hands.	____	____	_____
13. Reported and recorded observations.	____	____	_____

Date of Satisfactory Completion _____   Instructor's Initials _____

Measuring Blood Pressure

Name: _____   Date: _____

	S	U	Comments

Quality of Life

- Knocked before entering the person's room _____ _____ _____
- Addressed the person by name _____ _____ _____
- Introduced yourself by name and title _____ _____ _____

Pre-Procedure

1. Followed Delegation Guidelines. Reviewed Safety Alerts. _____ _____ _____
2. Collected the following:
   - Sphygmomanometer _____ _____ _____
   - Stethoscope _____ _____ _____
   - Antiseptic wipes _____ _____ _____
3. Practiced hand hygiene. _____ _____ _____
4. Identified the person. Checked the ID bracelet against the assignment sheet. Called the person by name. _____ _____ _____
5. Explained the procedure to the person. _____ _____ _____
6. Provided for privacy. _____ _____ _____

Procedure

7. Wiped the stethoscope earpieces and diaphragm with the wipes. _____ _____ _____
8. Had the person sit or lie down. _____ _____ _____
9. Positioned the person's arm level with the heart. The palm was up. _____ _____ _____
10. Stood no more than 3 feet away from the manometer. _____ _____ _____
11. Exposed the upper arm. _____ _____ _____
12. Squeezed the cuff to expel any remaining air. Closed the valve on the bulb. _____ _____ _____
13. Found the brachial artery at the inner aspect of the elbow. _____ _____ _____
14. Placed the arrow on the cuff over the brachial artery. Wrapped the cuff around the upper arm at least 1 inch above the elbow. It was even and snug. _____ _____ _____
15. *Method 1:*
    a. Placed the stethoscope earpieces in your ears. _____ _____ _____
    b. Found the radial or brachial artery. _____ _____ _____
    c. Inflated the cuff until the pulse could no longer be felt. Noted this point. _____ _____ _____
    d. Inflated the cuff 30 mm Hg beyond the point where the pulse was last felt. _____ _____ _____

    Method 2:
    e. Found the radial or brachial artery. _____ _____ _____
    f. Inflated the cuff until the pulse could no longer be felt. Noted this point. _____ _____ _____
    g. Inflated the cuff 30 mm Hg beyond the point where the pulse was last felt. _____ _____ _____

Procedure—cont'd   S   U   **Comments**

    h. Deflated the cuff slowly. Noted the point when the pulse was felt. ____ ____ _____

    i. Waited 30 seconds. ____ ____ _____

    j. Placed the stethoscope earpieces in your ears. ____ ____ _____

    k. Inflated the cuff 30 mm Hg beyond the point where you felt the pulse return. ____ ____ _____

16. Placed the diaphragm over the brachial artery. Did not place it under the cuff. ____ ____ _____

17. Deflated the cuff at an even rate of 2 to 4 millimeters per second. Turned the valve counterclockwise to deflate the cuff. ____ ____ _____

18. Noted the point where the first sound was heard. ____ ____ _____

19. Continued to deflate the cuff. Noted the point where the sound disappeared. ____ ____ _____

20. Deflated the cuff completely. Removed it from the person's arm. Removed the stethoscope. ____ ____ _____

21. Recorded the person's name and blood pressure on the note pad or assignment sheet. ____ ____ _____

22. Returned the cuff to the case or wall holder. ____ ____ _____

Post-Procedure

23. Provided for comfort. ____ ____ _____

24. Placed the signal light within reach. ____ ____ _____

25. Unscreened the person. ____ ____ _____

26. Completed a safety check of the room. ____ ____ _____

27. Cleaned the earpieces and diaphragm with the wipes. ____ ____ _____

28. Returned the equipment to its proper place. ____ ____ _____

29. Decontaminated hands. ____ ____ _____

30. Reported and recorded the blood pressure. ____ ____ _____

Date of Satisfactory Completion _____ Instructor's Initials _____

Measuring Height and Weight Using a Balance Scale

Name: _____   Date: _____

Quality of Life	S	U	Comments
• Knocked before entering the person's room	___	___	_____
• Addressed the person by name	___	___	_____
• Introduced yourself by name and title	___	___	_____

Pre-Procedure

	S	U	Comments
1. Followed Delegation Guidelines. Reviewed Safety Alert.	___	___	_____
2. Explained the procedure to the person.	___	___	_____
3. Asked the person to void.	___	___	_____
4. Practiced hand hygiene.	___	___	_____
5. Brought the balance or lift scale and paper towels to the person's room.	___	___	_____
6. Decontaminated hands.	___	___	_____
7. Identified the person. Checked the ID bracelet against the assignment sheet. Called the person by name.	___	___	_____
8. Provided for privacy.	___	___	_____

Procedure

	S	U	Comments
9. Placed the paper towels on the scale platform.	___	___	_____
10. Raised the height rod.	___	___	_____
11. Moved the weights to zero (0). The pointer was in the middle.	___	___	_____
12. Had the person remove the robe and footwear. Assisted as needed.	___	___	_____
13. Helped the person onto the scale.	___	___	_____
14. Moved the weights until the balance pointer was in the middle.	___	___	_____
15. Recorded the weight on the note pad or assignment sheet.	___	___	_____
16. Asked the person to stand very straight.	___	___	_____
17. Lowered the height rod until it rested on the person's head.	___	___	_____
18. Recorded the height on the note pad or assignment sheet.	___	___	_____
19. Helped the person put on a robe and nonskid footwear or helped the person back to bed.	___	___	_____

Post-Procedure

	S	U	Comments
20. Provided for comfort.	___	___	_____
21. Placed the signal light within reach.	___	___	_____
22. Raised or lowered bed rails. Followed the care plan.	___	___	_____
23. Unscreened the person.	___	___	_____
24. Discarded the paper towels.	___	___	_____
25. Completed a safety check of the room.	___	___	_____
26. Returned the scale to its proper place.	___	___	_____
27. Decontaminated hands.	___	___	_____
28. Reported and recorded the measurements.	___	___	_____

Date of Satisfactory Completion _____   Instructor's Initials _____

Measuring Intake and Output

Name: _____   Date: _____

Quality of Life	S	U	Comments
• Knocked before entering the person's room	____	____	_____
• Addressed the person by name	____	____	_____
• Introduced yourself by name and title	____	____	_____

Pre-Procedure

1. Followed Delegation Guidelines. Reviewed Safety Alert.   ____ ____ _____
2. Explained the procedure to the person.   ____ ____ _____
3. Practiced hand hygiene.   ____ ____ _____
4. Collected the following:
   - Intake and output (I&O) record   ____ ____ _____
   - Graduates   ____ ____ _____
   - Gloves   ____ ____ _____

Procedure

5. Practiced hand hygiene. Put on gloves.   ____ ____ _____
6. Measured intake as follows:
   a. Poured remaining liquid in a container into the graduate.   ____ ____ _____
   b. Measured the amount at eye level. Kept the container level.   ____ ____ _____
   c. Checked the serving amount on the I&O record.   ____ ____ _____
   d. Subtracted the remaining amount from the full serving amount. Recorded the amount.   ____ ____ _____
   e. Poured the fluid in the graduate back into the container.   ____ ____ _____
   f. Repeated steps 6a through 6e for each liquid.   ____ ____ _____
   g. Added the amounts from each liquid together.   ____ ____ _____
   h. Recorded the time and amount on the I&O record.   ____ ____ _____
7. Measured output as follows:
   a. Poured the fluid into the graduate used to measure output.   ____ ____ _____
   b. Measured the amount at eye level. Kept the container level.   ____ ____ _____
8. Disposed of fluid in the toilet. Avoided splashes.   ____ ____ _____
9. Cleaned and rinsed the graduate. Disposed of rinse into the toilet. Returned the graduate to its proper place.   ____ ____ _____
10. Cleaned and rinsed the bedpan, urinal, kidney basin, or other drainage container. Discarded the rinse into the toilet. Returned the item to its proper place.   ____ ____ _____
11. Removed the gloves. Decontaminated hands.   ____ ____ _____
12. Recorded the amount on the I&O record.   ____ ____ _____

Post-Procedure

13. Reported and recorded observations.   ____ ____ _____

Date of Satisfactory Completion _____   Instructor's Initials _____

Making a Closed Bed

Name: _____   Date: _____

Quality of Life	S	U	Comments
• Knocked before entering the person's room	____	____	_____
• Addressed the person by name	____	____	_____
• Introduced yourself by name and title	____	____	_____

Pre-Procedure

	S	U	Comments
1. Followed Delegation Guidelines. Reviewed Safety Alert.	____	____	_____
2. Practiced hand hygiene.	____	____	_____
3. Collected clean linen:			
• Mattress pad (if needed)	____	____	_____
• Bottom sheet (flat sheet or fitted sheet)	____	____	_____
• Plastic drawsheet or waterproof pad (if needed)	____	____	_____
• Cotton drawsheet (if needed)	____	____	_____
• Top sheet	____	____	_____
• Blanket	____	____	_____
• Bedspread	____	____	_____
• Two pillowcases	____	____	_____
• Bath towel(s)	____	____	_____
• Hand towel	____	____	_____
• Washcloth	____	____	_____
• Bath blanket	____	____	_____
• Gloves	____	____	_____
• Laundry bag	____	____	_____
4. Placed linen on a clean surface.	____	____	_____
5. Raised the bed for body mechanics.	____	____	_____

Procedure

	S	U	Comments
6. Put on the gloves.	____	____	_____
7. Removed linen. Rolled each piece away from you. Placed each piece in a laundry bag.	____	____	_____
8. Cleaned the bedframe and mattress if this is part of your job.	____	____	_____
9. Removed and discarded the gloves. Decontaminated hands.	____	____	_____
10. Moved the mattress to the head of the bed.	____	____	_____
11. Put the mattress pad on the mattress. It was even with the top of the mattress.	____	____	_____
12. Placed the bottom sheet on the mattress pad.	____	____	_____
a. Unfolded it lengthwise.	____	____	_____
b. Placed the center crease in the middle of the bed.	____	____	_____
c. Positioned the lower edge even with the bottom of the mattress.	____	____	_____

Procedure—cont'd

	S	U	Comments

d. Placed the large hem at the top and the small hem at the bottom.

e. Faced hem-stitching downward away from the person.

13. Opened the sheet. Fanfolded it to the other side of the bed.

14. Tucked the top of the sheet under the mattress. The sheet was tight and smooth.

15. Made a mitered corner if using a flat sheet.

16. Placed the plastic drawsheet on the bed about 14 inches from the top of the mattress. Or put the waterproof pad on the bed.

17. Opened the plastic drawsheet. Fanfolded it to the other side of the bed.

18. Placed a cotton drawsheet over the plastic drawsheet. It covered the entire plastic drawsheet.

19. Opened the cotton drawsheet. Fanfolded it to the other side of the bed.

20. Tucked both drawsheets under the mattress or tucked each in separately.

21. Went to the other side of the bed.

22. Mitered the top corner of the flat bottom sheet.

23. Pulled the bottom sheet tight so there were no wrinkles. Tucked in the sheet.

24. Pulled the drawsheets tight so there were no wrinkles. Tucked both in together or separately.

25. Went to the other side of the bed.

26. Put the top sheet on the bed.

   a. Unfolded it lengthwise.

   b. Placed the center crease in the middle.

   c. Placed the large hem even with the top of the mattress.

   d. Opened the sheet. Fanfolded it to the other side.

   e. Faced hem-stitching outward away from the person.

   f. Did not tuck the bottom in yet.

   g. Did not tuck top linens in on the sides.

27. Placed the blanket on the bed.

   a. Unfolded it so the center crease was in the middle.

   b. Put the upper hem about 6 to 8 inches from the top of the mattress.

   c. Opened the blanket. Fanfolded it to the other side.

   d. If steps 33 and 34 would not be done, turned the top sheet down over the blanket. Hem-stitching was down, away from the person.

28. Placed the bedspread on the bed.

   a. Unfolded it so the center crease was in the middle.

   b. Placed the upper hem even with the top of the mattress.

   c. Opened and fanfolded the spread to the other side.

Continued

Procedure—cont'd   S   U   **Comments**

    d. Made sure the spread facing the door was even. It covered all top linens.

29. Tucked in top linens together at the foot of the bed. They were smooth and tight. Made a mitered corner.

30. Went to the other side.

31. Straightened all top linen. Worked from the head of the bed to the foot.

32. Tucked in the top linens together at the foot of the bed. Made a mitered corner.

33. Turned the top hem of the spread under the blanket to make a cuff.

34. Turned the top sheet down over the spread. Hem-stitching was down. If steps 33 and 34 were not done, the spread covered the pillow and was tucked under the pillow.

35. Put the pillowcase on the pillow. Folded extra material under the pillow at the seam end of the pillowcase.

36. Placed the pillow on the bed. The open end was away from the door. The seam of the pillowcase was toward the head of the bed.

Post-Procedure

37. Attached the signal light to the bed.

38. Lowered the bed to its lowest position. Locked the bed wheels.

39. Put towels, washcloth, gown, and bath blanket in the bedside stand.

40. Completed a safety check of the room.

41. Followed center policy for dirty linen.

42. Decontaminated hands.

Date of Satisfactory Completion _____   Instructor's Initials _____

Making an Occupied Bed

Name: _____ Date: _____

Quality of Life	S	U	Comments
• Knocked before entering the person's room	____	____	_____
• Addressed the person by name	____	____	_____
• Introduced yourself by name and title	____	____	_____

Pre-Procedure

	S	U	Comments
1. Followed Delegation Guidelines. Reviewed Safety Alerts.	____	____	_____
2. Explained the procedure to the person.	____	____	_____
3. Practiced hand hygiene.	____	____	_____
4. Collected the following:			
a. Gloves	____	____	_____
b. Laundry bag	____	____	_____
c. Clean linen	____	____	_____
5. Placed linen on a clean surface.	____	____	_____
6. Identified the person. Checked the ID bracelet against the assignment sheet. Called the person by name.	____	____	_____
7. Provided for privacy.	____	____	_____
8. Removed the signal light.	____	____	_____
9. Raised the bed for body mechanics. Bed rails were up if used.	____	____	_____
10. Lowered the head of the bed. It was as flat as possible.	____	____	_____

Procedure

	S	U	Comments
11. Lowered the bed rail near you.	____	____	_____
12. Practiced hand hygiene. Put on gloves.	____	____	_____
13. Loosened top linens at the foot of the bed.	____	____	_____
14. Removed the bedspread. Then removed the blanket. Placed each over the chair.	____	____	_____
15. Covered the person with a bath blanket.	____	____	_____
a. Unfolded a bath blanket over the top sheet.	____	____	_____
b. Asked the person to hold onto the bath blanket. If the person could not, tucked the top part under the person's shoulders.	____	____	_____
c. Grasped the top sheet under the bath blanket at the shoulders. Brought the sheet down to the foot of the bed. Removed the sheet from under the blanket.	____	____	_____
16. Moved the mattress to the head of the bed (optional).	____	____	_____
17. Positioned the person on the side of the bed away from you. Adjusted the pillow for comfort.	____	____	_____
18. Loosened bottom linens from the head to the foot of the bed.	____	____	_____
19. Fanfolded bottom linens one at a time toward the person. Started with the cotton drawsheet. If reusing the mattress pad, did not fanfold it.	____	____	_____

Continued

Procedure—cont'd

	S	U	Comments

20. Placed a clean mattress pad on the bed. Unfolded it lengthwise. The center crease was in the middle. Fanfolded the top part toward the person. If reusing the mattress pad, straightened it and removed any wrinkles.

21. Placed the bottom sheet on the mattress pad. Hem-stitching was away from the person. Unfolded the sheet so the crease was in the middle. The small hem was even with the bottom of the mattress. Fanfolded the top part toward the person.

22. Made a mitered corner at the head of the bed. Tucked the sheet under the mattress from the head to the foot.

23. Pulled the plastic drawsheet toward you over the bottom sheet. Tucked excess material under the mattress. Did the following for a clean plastic drawsheet:

    a. Placed the plastic drawsheet on the bed. It was about 14 inches from the mattress top.

    b. Fanfolded the top part toward the person.

    c. Tucked in the excess fabric.

24. Placed the cotton drawsheet over the plastic drawsheet. Fanfolded the top part toward the person. Tucked in excess fabric.

25. Raised the bed rail if used. Went to the other side and lowered the bed rail.

26. Explained to the person that he or she would roll over a bump. Assured the person that he or she would not fall.

27. Helped the person turn to the other side. Adjusted the pillow for comfort.

28. Loosened bottom linens. Removed one piece at a time. Placed each piece in the laundry bag.

29. Removed and discarded the gloves. Decontaminated your hands.

30. Straightened and smoothed the mattress pad.

31. Pulled the clean bottom sheet toward you. Made a mitered corner at the top. Tucked the sheet under the mattress from the head to the foot of the bed.

32. Pulled the drawsheets tightly toward you. Tucked both under together or separately.

33. Positioned the person supine in the center of the bed. Adjusted the pillow for comfort.

34. Put the top sheet on the bed. Unfolded it lengthwise. The crease was in the middle. The large hem was even with the top of the mattress. Hem-stitching was on the outside.

35. Asked the person to hold onto the top sheet or tuck the top sheet under the person's shoulders. Removed the bath blanket.

36. Placed the blanket on the bed. Unfolded it so the crease was in the middle and it covered the person. The upper hem was 6 to 8 inches from the top of the mattress.

37. Placed the bedspread on the bed. Unfolded it so the center crease was in the middle and it covered the person. The top hem was even with the mattress top.

Procedure—cont'd	S	U	Comments
38. Turned the top hem of the spread under the blanket to make a cuff.	____	____	_____
39. Brought the top sheet down over the spread to form a cuff.	____	____	_____
40. Went to the foot of the bed.	____	____	_____
41. Made a 2-inch toe pleat about 6 to 8 inches from the foot of the bed.	____	____	_____
42. Lifted the mattress corner with one arm. Tucked all top linens under the mattress together. Made a mitered corner.	____	____	_____
43. Raised the bed rail if used. Went to the other side and lowered the bed rail if used.	____	____	_____
44. Straightened and smoothed top linens.	____	____	_____
45. Tucked the top linens under the mattress. Made a mitered corner.	____	____	_____
46. Changed the pillowcase(s).	____	____	_____

Post-Procedure

	S	U	Comments
47. Placed the signal light within reach.	____	____	_____
48. Raised or lowered bed rails. Followed the care plan.	____	____	_____
49. Raised the head of the bed to a level appropriate for the person. Provided for comfort.	____	____	_____
50. Lowered the bed to its lowest position. Locked the bed wheels.	____	____	_____
51. Put towels, washcloth, and bath blanket in the bedside stand.	____	____	_____
52. Unscreened the person.	____	____	_____
53. Completed a safety check of the room.	____	____	_____
54. Followed center policy for dirty linen.	____	____	_____
55. Decontaminated hands.	____	____	_____

Date of Satisfactory Completion _____ Instructor's Initials _____

Assisting With Postmortem Care

Name: _____   Date: _____

Pre-Procedure

	S	U	Comments

1. Followed Delegation Guidelines. Reviewed Safety Alert. _____ _____ _____
2. Practiced hand hygiene. _____ _____ _____
3. Collected the following:
   - Postmortem kit (shroud or body bag, gown, ID tags, gauze squares, safety pins) _____ _____ _____
   - Bed protectors _____ _____ _____
   - Washbasin _____ _____ _____
   - Bath towels and washcloths _____ _____ _____
   - Denture cup if needed _____ _____ _____
   - Tape _____ _____ _____
   - Dressings _____ _____ _____
   - Gloves _____ _____ _____
   - Cotton balls _____ _____ _____
   - Gown _____ _____ _____
   - Valuables envelope _____ _____ _____
4. Provided for privacy. _____ _____ _____
5. Raised the bed for body mechanics. _____ _____ _____
6. Made sure the bed was flat. _____ _____ _____

Procedure

7. Put on the gloves. _____ _____ _____
8. Positioned the body supine. Arms and legs were straight. A pillow was under the head and shoulders. _____ _____ _____
9. Closed the eyes. Gently pulled the eyelids over the eyes. Applied moist cotton balls gently over the eyelids if the eyes would not stay closed. _____ _____ _____
10. Inserted dentures if it was center policy. If not, put them in a labeled denture cup. _____ _____ _____
11. Closed the mouth. If necessary, placed a rolled towel under the chin to keep the mouth closed. _____ _____ _____
12. Followed center policy about jewelry. Removed all jewelry, except for wedding rings if this was center policy. Listed the jewelry that was removed. Placed the jewelry and the list in a valuables envelope. _____ _____ _____
13. Placed a cotton ball over the rings. Taped them in place. _____ _____ _____

Procedure—cont'd

	S	U	Comments

14. Removed drainage containers. Left tubes and catheters in place if there would be an autopsy. Asked the nurse about removing tubes.

15. Bathed soiled areas with plain water. Dried thoroughly.

16. Placed a bed protector under the buttocks.

17. Removed soiled dressings. Replaced them with clean ones.

18. Put a clean gown on the body. Positioned the body as in step 8.

19. Brushed and combed the hair if necessary.

20. Covered the body to the shoulders with a sheet if the family would view the body.

21. Gathered the person's belongings. Put them in a bag labeled with the person's name.

22. Removed supplies, equipment, and linen. Straightened the room. Provided soft lighting.

23. Removed the gloves. Decontaminated hands.

24. Let the family view the body. Provided for privacy. Returned to the room after they left.

25. Decontaminated hands. Put on gloves.

26. Filled out the ID tags. Tied one to the ankle or to the right big toe.

27. Placed the body in the body bag or covered it with a sheet, or applied the shroud.
    a. Brought the top down over the head.
    b. Folded the bottom up over the feet.
    c. Folded the sides over the body.
    d. Pinned or taped the shroud in place.

28. Attached the second ID tag to the shroud, sheet, or body bag.

29. Left the denture cup with the body.

30. Pulled the privacy curtain around the bed or closed the door.

Post-Procedure

31. Removed the gloves. Decontaminated hands.

32. Stripped the unit after the body was removed. Wore gloves for this step.

33. Removed the gloves. Decontaminated hands.

34. Reported the following to the nurse:
    • The time the body was taken by the funeral director
    • What was done with jewelry and personal items
    • What was done with dentures

Date of Satisfactory Completion _____ Instructor's Initials _____

Brushing the Person's Teeth

Name: _____   Date: _____

Quality of Life	S	U	Comments
• Knocked before entering the person's room	___	___	_____
• Addressed the person by name	___	___	_____
• Introduced yourself by name and title	___	___	_____

Pre-Procedure

	S	U	Comments
1. Followed Delegation Guidelines. Reviewed Safety Alert.	___	___	_____
2. Explained the procedure to the person.	___	___	_____
3. Practiced hand hygiene.	___	___	_____
4. Collected the following:			
• Toothbrush	___	___	_____
• Toothpaste	___	___	_____
• Mouthwash or solution on care plan	___	___	_____
• Water glass with cool water	___	___	_____
• Straw	___	___	_____
• Kidney basin	___	___	_____
• Hand towel	___	___	_____
• Paper towels	___	___	_____
• Gloves	___	___	_____
5. Placed the paper towels on the overbed table. Arranged items on top of them.	___	___	_____
6. Identified the person. Checked the ID bracelet against the assignment sheet. Called the person by name.	___	___	_____
7. Provided for privacy.	___	___	_____
8. Raised the bed for body mechanics. Bed rails were up if used.	___	___	_____

Procedure

	S	U	Comments
9. Lowered the bed rail near you if up.	___	___	_____
10. Assisted the person to a sitting position or to a side-lying position near you.	___	___	_____
11. Placed the towel over the person's chest.	___	___	_____
12. Adjusted the overbed table so it could be reached with ease.	___	___	_____
13. Decontaminated hands. Put on the gloves.	___	___	_____
14. Applied toothpaste to the toothbrush.	___	___	_____
15. Held the toothbrush over the kidney basin. Poured some water over the brush.	___	___	_____
16. Brushed the teeth gently.	___	___	_____
17. Brushed the tongue gently.	___	___	_____
18. Let the person rinse the mouth with water. Held the kidney basin under the person's chin. Repeated this step as needed.	___	___	_____
19. Let the person use mouthwash or other solution. Held the kidney basin under the chin.	___	___	_____

Procedure—cont'd	S	U	Comments
20. Wiped the person's mouth and removed the towel.	_____	_____	_____
21. Removed and discarded the gloves. Decontaminated hands.	_____	_____	_____

Post-Procedure

	S	U	Comments
22. Provided for comfort.	_____	_____	_____
23. Placed the signal light within reach.	_____	_____	_____
24. Lowered the bed to its lowest position.	_____	_____	_____
25. Raised or lowered bed rails. Follow the care plan.	_____	_____	_____
26. Cleaned and return equipment to its proper place. Wore gloves.	_____	_____	_____
27. Wiped off the overbed table with the paper towels. Discarded the paper towels.	_____	_____	_____
28. Removed the gloves. Decontaminated hands.	_____	_____	_____
29. Adjusted the overbed table for the person.	_____	_____	_____
30. Unscreened the person.	_____	_____	_____
31. Completed a safety check of the room.	_____	_____	_____
32. Followed center policy for dirty linen.	_____	_____	_____
33. Decontaminated hands.	_____	_____	_____
34. Reported and recorded observations.	_____	_____	_____

Date of Satisfactory Completion _____ Instructor's Initials _____

Providing Mouth Care for the Unconscious Person

Name: _____   Date: _____

Quality of Life	**S**	**U**	**Comments**

- Knocked before entering the person's room
- Addressed the person by name
- Introduced yourself by name and title

Pre-Procedure

1. Followed Delegation Guidelines. Reviewed Safety Alert.
2. Practiced hand hygiene.
3. Collected the following:
   - Cleaning agent
   - Sponge swabs
   - Padded tongue blade
   - Water glass with cool water
   - Hand towel
   - Kidney basin
   - Lip lubricant
   - Paper towels
   - Gloves
4. Placed the paper towels on the overbed table. Arranged items on top of them.
5. Identified the person. Checked the ID bracelet against the assignment sheet. Called the person by name.
6. Explained the procedure to the person.
7. Provided for privacy.
8. Raised the bed for body mechanics. Bed rails were up if used.

Procedure

9. Lowered the bed rail near you if up.
10. Decontaminated hands. Put on the gloves.
11. Positioned the person in a side-lying position near you. Turned the person's head well to the side.
12. Placed the towel under the person's face.
13. Placed the kidney basin under the chin.
14. Adjusted the overbed table so it could be reached with ease.
15. Separated the upper and lower teeth. Used the padded tongue blade. Did not use force. Asked the nurse for help if needed.
16. Cleaned the mouth using sponge swabs moistened with the cleaning agent.
    a. Cleaned the chewing and inner surfaces of the teeth.
    b. Cleaned the outer surfaces of the teeth.
    c. Swabbed the roof of the mouth, inside of the cheeks, and the lips.

Procedure—cont'd   S   U   Comments

    d. Swabbed the tongue.

    e. Moistened a clean swab with water. Swabbed the mouth to rinse.

    f. Placed used swabs in the kidney basin.

17. Applied lubricant to the lips.

18. Wiped the person's mouth and removed the towel.

19. Removed and discarded the gloves. Decontaminated hands.

20. Explained that the procedure was done. Explained that you would reposition the person.

21. Repositioned the person. Provided for comfort.

22. Raised or lower bed rails. Followed the care plan.

Post-Procedure

23. Placed the signal light within reach.

24. Lowered the bed to its lowest position.

25. Cleaned and returned equipment to its proper place. Discarded disposable items. Wore gloves.

26. Wiped off the overbed table with paper towels. Discarded the paper towels.

27. Removed the gloves. Decontaminated hands.

28. Unscreened the person.

29. Completed a safety check of the room.

30. Told the person that you were leaving the room.

31. Followed center policy for dirty linen.

32. Decontaminated hands.

33. Reported and recorded observations.

Date of Satisfactory Completion _____   Instructor's Initials _____

Providing Denture Care

Name: _____   Date: _____

Quality of Life	S	U	Comments
• Knocked before entering the person's room	_____	_____	_____
• Addressed the person by name	_____	_____	_____
• Introduced yourself by name and title	_____	_____	_____

Pre-Procedure

1. Followed Delegation Guidelines. Reviewed Safety Alerts. _____ _____ _____
2. Explained the procedure to the person. _____ _____ _____
3. Practiced hand hygiene. _____ _____ _____
4. Collected the following:
   • Denture brush or soft-bristled toothbrush _____ _____ _____
   • Denture cup labeled with the person's name and room number _____ _____ _____
   • Cleaning agent _____ _____ _____
   • Water glass with cool water _____ _____ _____
   • Straw _____ _____ _____
   • Mouthwash or other noted solution _____ _____ _____
   • Kidney basin _____ _____ _____
   • Two hand towels _____ _____ _____
   • Gauze squares _____ _____ _____
   • Gloves _____ _____ _____
5. Identified the person. Checked the ID bracelet against the assignment sheet. Called the person by name. _____ _____ _____
6. Provided for privacy. _____ _____ _____

Procedure

7. Lowered the bed rail near you if used. _____ _____ _____
8. Placed a towel over the person's chest. _____ _____ _____
9. Decontaminated hands. Put on the gloves. _____ _____ _____
10. Asked the person to remove the dentures. Carefully placed them in the kidney basin. _____ _____ _____
11. Removed the dentures if the person could not do so. Used gauze squares to get a good grip on the dentures. _____ _____ _____
    a. Grasped the upper denture with the thumb and index finger. Moved it up and down slightly to break the seal. Gently removed the denture. Placed it in the kidney basin. _____ _____ _____
    b. Grasped and removed the lower denture with the thumb and index finger. Turned it slightly and lifted it out of the mouth. Placed it in the kidney basin. _____ _____ _____
12. Followed the care plan for raising bed rails. _____ _____ _____
13. Took the kidney basin, denture cup, brush, and cleaning agent to the sink. _____ _____ _____

Procedure—cont'd	**S**	**U**	**Comments**
14. Lined the sink with a towel. Filled the sink with water until it was half full.	___	___	_____
15. Rinsed each denture under warm or cool running water. Rinsed out the denture cup.	___	___	_____
16. Returned dentures to the denture cup.	___	___	_____
17. Applied the cleaning agent to the brush.	___	___	_____
18. Brushed the dentures.	___	___	_____
19. Rinsed dentures under running water. Used warm or cool water as directed by the cleaning agent manufacturer.	___	___	_____
20. Rinsed the denture cup. Placed dentures in the denture cup. Covered the dentures with cool water.	___	___	_____
21. Cleaned the kidney basin.	___	___	_____
22. Took the denture cup and kidney basin to the bedside table.	___	___	_____
23. Lowered the bed rail if up.	___	___	_____
24. Positioned the person for oral hygiene.	___	___	_____
25. Had the person use mouthwash or noted solution. Held the kidney basin under the chin.	___	___	_____
26. Asked the person to insert the dentures. Inserted them if the person could not.	___	___	_____
a. Held the upper denture firmly with the thumb and index finger. Raised the upper lip with the other hand. Inserted the denture. Gently pressed on the denture with the index fingers to make sure it was in place.	___	___	_____
b. Held the lower denture with the thumb and index finger. Pulled the lower lip down slightly. Inserted the denture. Gently pressed down on it to make sure it was in place.	___	___	_____
27. Placed the denture cup in the top drawer of the bedside stand if the dentures were not worn. The dentures must be in water or in a denture soaking solution.	___	___	_____
28. Wiped the person's mouth and removed the towel.	___	___	_____
29. Removed the gloves. Decontaminated hands.	___	___	_____

Post-Procedure

	S	**U**	**Comments**
30. Assisted with hand washing.	___	___	_____
31. Provided for comfort.	___	___	_____
32. Placed the signal light within reach.	___	___	_____
33. Raised or lowered bed rails. Followed the care plan.	___	___	_____
34. Unscreened the person.	___	___	_____
35. Cleaned and returned equipment to its proper place. Discarded disposable items. Wore gloves for this step.	___	___	_____
36. Completed a safety check of the room.	___	___	_____
37. Followed center policy for dirty linen.	___	___	_____
38. Decontaminated hands.	___	___	_____
39. Reported and recorded observations.	___	___	_____

Date of Satisfactory Completion _____ Instructor's Initials _____

Giving a Complete Bed Bath

Name: _____   Date: _____

Quality of Life	**S**	**U**	**Comments**

- Knocked before entering the person's room   _____ _____ _____
- Addressed the person by name   _____ _____ _____
- Introduced yourself by name and title   _____ _____ _____

Pre-Procedure

1. Followed Delegation Guidelines. Reviewed Safety Alert.   _____ _____ _____
2. Practiced hand hygiene   _____ _____ _____
3. Identified the person. Checked the ID bracelet against the assignment sheet. Called the person by name.   _____ _____ _____
4. Explained the procedure to the person.   _____ _____ _____
5. Offered the bedpan or urinal. Provided for privacy.   _____ _____ _____
6. Collected clean linen for a closed bed. Placed linen on a clean surface.   _____ _____ _____
7. Collected the following:
   - Wash basin   _____ _____ _____
   - Soap   _____ _____ _____
   - Bath thermometer   _____ _____ _____
   - Orange stick or nail file   _____ _____ _____
   - Washcloth   _____ _____ _____
   - Two bath towels and two hand towels   _____ _____ _____
   - Bath blanket   _____ _____ _____
   - Clothing, gown, or pajamas   _____ _____ _____
   - Items for oral hygiene   _____ _____ _____
   - Lotion   _____ _____ _____
   - Powder   _____ _____ _____
   - Deodorant or antiperspirant   _____ _____ _____
   - Brush and comb   _____ _____ _____
   - Other grooming items if requested   _____ _____ _____
   - Paper towels   _____ _____ _____
   - Gloves   _____ _____ _____
8. Arranged items on the overbed table. Adjusted the height as needed.   _____ _____ _____
9. Closed doors and windows to prevent drafts.   _____ _____ _____
10. Provided for privacy.   _____ _____ _____
11. Raised the bed for body mechanics. Bed rails were up if used.   _____ _____ _____

Procedure

12. Removed the signal light. Lowered the bed rail near you if up.   _____ _____ _____
13. Decontaminated hands. Put on gloves.   _____ _____ _____
14. Provided oral hygiene.   _____ _____ _____

Procedure—cont'd   S   U   Comments

15. Covered the person with a bath blanket. Removed top linens. (See procedure: Making an Occupied Bed.)   ____ ____ _____

16. Lowered the head of the bed. It was as flat as possible. The person had at least one pillow.   ____ ____ _____

17. Covered the overbed table with paper towels.   ____ ____ _____

18. Raised the bed rail near you if bed rails are used. Both bed rails must be up.   ____ ____ _____

19. Filled the wash basin ⅔ full with water. Measured water temperature. Used a bath thermometer or tested the water by dipping the elbow or inner wrist into the basin.   ____ ____ _____

20. Placed the basin on the overbed table.   ____ ____ _____

21. Lowered the bed rail if up.   ____ ____ _____

22. Placed a hand towel over the person's chest.   ____ ____ _____

23. Made a mitt with the washcloth. Used a mitt for the entire bath.   ____ ____ _____

24. Washed around the person's eyes with water. Did not use soap. Gently wiped from the inner to the outer aspect of the eyelid with a corner of the mitt. Cleaned the far eye first. Repeated this step for the near eye. Used a clean part of the washcloth for each stroke.   ____ ____ _____

25. Asked the person if you should use soap to wash the face.   ____ ____ _____

26. Washed the face, ears, and neck. Rinsed and patted dry with the towel on the chest.   ____ ____ _____

27. Helped the person move to the side of the bed near you.   ____ ____ _____

28. Removed the gown. Did not expose the person.   ____ ____ _____

29. Placed a bath towel lengthwise under the far arm.   ____ ____ _____

30. Supported the arm with your palm under the person's elbow. The person's forearm rested on your forearm.   ____ ____ _____

31. Washed the arm, shoulder, and underarm. Used long, firm strokes. Rinsed and patted dry.   ____ ____ _____

32. Placed the basin on the towel. Put the person's hand into the water. Washed it well. Cleaned under fingernails with an orange stick or nail file.   ____ ____ _____

33. Removed the basin. Dried the hand well. Covered the arm with the bath blanket.   ____ ____ _____

34. Repeated steps 29 to 33 for the near arm.   ____ ____ _____

35. Placed a bath towel over the chest crosswise. Held the towel in place. Pulled the bath blanket from under the towel to the waist.   ____ ____ _____

36. Lifted the towel slightly and washed the chest. Did not expose the person. Rinsed and patted dry especially under breasts.   ____ ____ _____

37. Moved the towel lengthwise over the chest and abdomen. Did not expose the person. Pulled the bath blanket down to the pubic area.   ____ ____ _____

38. Lifted the towel slightly and washed the abdomen. Rinsed and patted dry.   ____ ____ _____

39. Pulled the bath blanket up to the shoulders, covering both arms. Removed the towel.   ____ ____ _____

Continued

Procedure—cont'd

	S	U	Comments

40. Changed soapy or cool water. Measured bath water as in step 19. If bed rails were used, raised the bed rail near you before leaving the bedside. Lowered it when you returned.

41. Uncovered the far leg. Did not expose the genital area. Placed a towel lengthwise under the foot and leg.

42. Bent the knee and supported the leg with your arm. Washed it with long, firm strokes. Rinsed and patted dry.

43. Placed the basin on the towel near the foot.

44. Lifted the leg slightly. Slid the basin under the foot.

45. Placed the foot in the basin. Used an orange stick or nail file to clean under toenails if necessary. If the person could not bend the knees:

    a. Washed the foot. Carefully separated the toes. Rinsed and patted dry.

    b. Cleaned under the toenails with an orange stick or nail file if necessary.

46. Removed the basin. Dried the leg and foot. Covered the leg with the bath blanket. Removed the towel.

47. Repeated steps 41 to 46 for the near leg.

48. Changed the water. Measured bath water as in step 19. If bed rails were used, raised the bed rail near you before leaving the bedside. Lowered it when you returned.

49. Turned the person onto the side away from you.

50. Uncovered the back and buttocks. Did not expose the person. Placed a towel lengthwise on the bed along the back.

51. Washed the back. Worked from the back of the neck to the lower end of the buttocks. Used long, firm, continuous strokes. Rinsed and dried well.

52. Turned the person onto his or her back.

53. Changed the water for perineal care. Measured bath water as in step 19. Changed gloves and practiced hand hygiene if required. If bed rails were used, raised the bed rail near you before leaving the bedside. Lowered it when you returned.

54. Let the person wash the genital area. Adjusted the overbed table so the person could reach the wash basin, soap, and towels with ease. Placed the signal light within reach. Asked the person to signal when finished. Made sure the person understood what to do.

55. Removed the gloves. Decontaminated hands.

56. Answered the signal light promptly. Provided perineal care if the person could not do so. Decontaminated hands and wore gloves for perineal care.

57. Gave a back massage.

58. Applied deodorant or antiperspirant. Applied lotion and powder as requested.

59. Put clean garments on the person.

60. Combed and brushed the hair.

61. Made the bed. Attached the signal light.

Post-Procedure

	S	U	Comments
62. Provided for comfort.	_____	_____	_____
63. Lowered the bed to its lowest position.	_____	_____	_____
64. Raised or lowered bed rails. Followed the care plan.	_____	_____	_____
65. Put on gloves.	_____	_____	_____
66. Emptied and cleaned the wash basin. Returned it and other supplies to their proper place.	_____	_____	_____
67. Wiped off the overbed table with the paper towels. Discarded the paper towels.	_____	_____	_____
68. Unscreened the person.	_____	_____	_____
69. Completed a safety check of the room.	_____	_____	_____
70. Followed center policy for dirty linen.	_____	_____	_____
71. Removed the gloves. Decontaminated hands.	_____	_____	_____
72. Reported and recorded observations.	_____	_____	_____

Date of Satisfactory Completion _____ Instructor's Initials _____

Giving a Partial Bath

Name: _____ Date: _____

	S	U	Comments

Quality of Life

- Knocked before entering the person's room
- Addressed the person by name
- Introduced yourself by name and title

Pre-Procedure

1. Followed Delegation Guidelines. Reviewed Safety Alert.
2. Followed steps 2 through 10 in procedure: Giving a Complete Bed Bath.

Procedure

3. Made sure the bed was in the lowest position.
4. Assisted with oral hygiene. Wore gloves.
5. Removed top linen. Covered the person with a bath blanket.
6. Covered the overbed table with paper towels.
7. Filled the wash basin $2/3$ full with water. Measured water temperature with the bath thermometer or tested bath water by dipping the elbow or inner wrist into the basin.
8. Placed the basin on the overbed table.
9. Positioned the person in Fowler's position or assisted the person to sit at the bedside.
10. Adjusted the overbed table so the person could reach the basin and supplies.
11. Helped the person undress.
12. Asked the person to wash easy-to-reach body parts. Explained that you would wash the back and areas the person could not reach.
13. Placed the signal light within reach. Asked the person to signal when help was needed or bathing was complete.
14. Left the room after decontaminating hands.
15. Returned when the signal light was on. Knocked before entering. Decontaminated hands.
16. Changed the bath water. Measured bath water temperature as in step 7.
17. Raised the bed for body mechanics. The far bed rail was up if used.
18. Asked what was washed. Put on gloves. Washed and dried areas the person could not reach. The face, hands, underarms, back, buttocks, and perineal area were washed for the partial bath.
19. Removed the gloves. Decontaminated hands.
20. Gave a back massage.
21. Applied lotion, powder, and deodorant or antiperspirant as requested.

Procedure—cont'd   **S**   **U**   **Comments**

22. Helped the person put on clean garments.   _____ _____ _____

23. Assisted with hair care and other grooming needs.   _____ _____ _____

24. Assisted the person to a chair. (Lowered the bed if the person transfers to a chair.) Otherwise, turned the person onto the side away from you.   _____ _____ _____

25. Made the bed.   _____ _____ _____

26. Lowered the bed to its lowest position.   _____ _____ _____

Post-Procedure

27. Provided for comfort.   _____ _____ _____

28. Placed the signal light within reach.   _____ _____ _____

29. Raised or lowered bed rails. Followed the care plan.   _____ _____ _____

30. Put on gloves.   _____ _____ _____

31. Emptied and cleaned the basin. Returned the basin and supplies to their proper place.   _____ _____ _____

32. Wiped off the overbed table with the paper towels. Discarded the paper towels.   _____ _____ _____

33. Unscreened the person.   _____ _____ _____

34. Completed a safety check of the room.   _____ _____ _____

35. Followed center policy for dirty linen.   _____ _____ _____

36. Removed the gloves. Decontaminated hands.   _____ _____ _____

37. Reported and recorded observations.   _____ _____ _____

Date of Satisfactory Completion _____ Instructor's Initials _____

Assisting With a Tub Bath or Shower

Name: _____ Date: _____

Quality of Life	S	U	Comments

- Knocked before entering the person's room
- Addressed the person by name
- Introduced yourself by name and title

Pre-Procedure

1. Followed Delegation Guidelines. Reviewed Safety Alert.
2. Reserved the bathtub or shower.
3. Practiced hand hygiene.
4. Identified the person. Checked the ID bracelet against the assignment sheet. Called the person by name.
5. Explained the procedure to the person.
6. Collected the following:
   - Washcloth and two bath towels
   - Soap
   - Bath thermometer (for a tub bath)
   - Clothing, gown, or pajamas
   - Grooming items as requested
   - Robe and nonskid footwear
   - Rubber bath mat if needed
   - Disposable bath mat
   - Gloves
   - Wheelchair or shower chair

Procedure

7. Placed items in the tub or shower room. Used the space provided or a chair.
8. Cleaned and disinfected the tub or shower.
9. Placed a rubber bath mat in the tub or on the shower floor. Did not block the drain.
10. Placed a disposable bath mat on the floor in front of tub or shower.
11. Put the "Occupied" sign on the door.
12. Returned to the person's room. Decontaminated hands.
13. Provided for privacy.
14. Helped the person sit on the side of the bed.
15. Helped the person put on a robe and nonskid footwear.
16. Assisted or transported the person to the tub or shower room.
17. Had the person sit on the chair. Provided for privacy.
18. For a tub bath:
    a. Filled the tub halfway with warm water (105° F; 41° C). Measured water temperature with the bath thermometer or checked the digital display.

Procedure—cont'd   S   U   Comments

19. For a shower:
   a. Turned on the shower. _____ _____ _____
   b. Adjusted water temperature and pressure. _____ _____ _____
20. Helped the person undress and remove footwear. _____ _____ _____
21. Helped the person into the tub or shower. Positioned the shower chair and locked the wheels. _____ _____ _____
22. Assisted with washing if necessary. Wore gloves. _____ _____ _____
23. Asked the person to use the signal light when done or when help was needed. Reminded the person that a tub bath lasts no longer than 20 minutes. _____ _____ _____
24. Placed a towel across the chair. _____ _____ _____
25. Left the room if the person could bathe unattended. If not, stayed in the room or remained nearby. Removed the gloves and decontaminated hands if you left the room. _____ _____ _____
26. Checked the person every 5 minutes. _____ _____ _____
27. Returned when the person signaled. Knocked before entering. Decontaminated hands. _____ _____ _____
28. Turned off the shower or drained the tub. Covered the person while the tub drained. _____ _____ _____
29. Helped the person out of the tub or shower and onto the chair. _____ _____ _____
30. Helped the person dry off. Patted gently. Dried under breasts, between skin folds, in the perineal area, and between the toes. _____ _____ _____
31. Assisted with lotion and other grooming items as needed. _____ _____ _____
32. Helped the person dress and put on footwear. _____ _____ _____
33. Helped the person return to the room. Provided for privacy. _____ _____ _____
34. Assisted the person to a chair or into bed. _____ _____ _____
35. Provided a back massage. _____ _____ _____
36. Assisted with hair care and other grooming needs. _____ _____ _____

Post-Procedure

37. Made the bed. Provided for comfort. _____ _____ _____
38. Raised or lowered bed rails. Followed the care plan. _____ _____ _____
39. Placed the signal light within reach. _____ _____ _____
40. Unscreened the person. _____ _____ _____
41. Completed a safety check of the room. _____ _____ _____
42. Cleaned and disinfected the tub or shower. Removed soiled linen. Wore gloves for this step. _____ _____ _____
43. Discarded disposable items. Put the "Unoccupied" sign on the door. Returned supplies to their proper place. _____ _____ _____
44. Followed center policy for dirty linen. _____ _____ _____
45. Decontaminated hands. _____ _____ _____
46. Reported and recorded observations. _____ _____ _____

Date of Satisfactory Completion _____   Instructor's Initials _____

Giving a Back Massage

Name: _____   Date: _____

Quality of Life	S	U	Comments

Quality of Life

- Knocked before entering the person's room
- Addressed the person by name
- Introduced yourself by name and title

Pre-Procedure

1. Followed Delegation Guidelines. Reviewed Safety Alert.
2. Practiced hand hygiene.
3. Identified the person. Checked the ID bracelet against the assignment sheet. Called the person by name.
4. Explained the procedure to the person.
5. Collected the following:
   - Bath blanket
   - Bath towel
   - Lotion
6. Provided for privacy.
7. Raised the bed for body mechanics. Bed rails were up if used.

Procedure

8. Lowered the bed rail near you if up.
9. Positioned the person in the prone or side-lying position with the back toward you.
10. Exposed the back, shoulders, upper arms, and buttocks. Covered the rest of the body with the bath blanket.
11. Laid the towel on the bed along the back.
12. Warmed the lotion.
13. Applied lotion to the lower back area.
14. Stroked up from the buttocks to the shoulders. Then stroked down over the upper arms. Stroked up the upper arms, across the shoulders, and down the back to the buttocks. Used firm strokes. Kept hands in contact with the person's skin.
15. Repeated Step 14 for at least 3 minutes.
16. Kneaded by grasping skin between the thumb and fingers. Kneaded half of the back. Started at the buttocks and moved up to the shoulder. Then kneaded down from the shoulder to the buttocks. Repeated on the other half of the back.
17. Applied lotion to bony areas. Used circular motions with the tips of the index and middle fingers. Did not massage reddened bony areas.
18. Used fast movements to stimulate. Used slow movements to relax the person.
19. Stroked with long, firm movements to end the massage. Told the person you were finishing.

Post-Procedure   S   U   Comments

20. Covered the person. Removed the towel and bath blanket.   _____ _____ _____

21. Provided for comfort.   _____ _____ _____

22. Lowered the bed to its lowest position.   _____ _____ _____

23. Raised or lowered bed rails. Followed the care plan.   _____ _____ _____

24. Placed the signal light within reach.   _____ _____ _____

25. Returned lotion to its proper place.   _____ _____ _____

26. Unscreened the person.   _____ _____ _____

27. Completed a safety check of the room.   _____ _____ _____

28. Followed center policy for dirty linen.   _____ _____ _____

29. Decontaminated hands.   _____ _____ _____

30. Reported and recorded observations.   _____ _____ _____

Date of Satisfactory Completion _____ Instructor's Initials _____

Giving Perineal Care

Name: _____   Date: _____

Quality of Life

	S	U	Comments

- Knocked before entering the person's room
- Addressed the person by name
- Introduced yourself by name and title

Pre-Procedure

1. Followed Delegation Guidelines. Reviewed Safety Alert.
2. Explained the procedure to the person.
3. Practiced hand hygiene.
4. Collected the following:
   - Soap
   - At least 4 washcloths
   - Bath towel
   - Bath blanket
   - Bath thermometer
   - Washbasin
   - Waterproof pad
   - Gloves
   - Paper towels
5. Covered the overbed table with paper towels. Arranged items on top of them.
6. Identified the person. Checked the ID bracelet against the assignment sheet. Called the person by name.
7. Provided for privacy.
8. Raised the bed for body mechanics. Bed rails were up if used.

Procedure

9. Lowered the bed rail near you if up.
10. Covered the person with a bath blanket. Moved top linens to the foot of the bed.
11. Positioned the person supine.
12. Draped the person.
13. Raised the bed rail if used.
14. Filled the wash basin $2/3$ full with water. Measured water temperature according to center policy.
15. Placed the basin on the overbed table.
16. Lowered the bed rail if up.
17. Decontaminated hands. Put on the gloves.
18. Helped the person flex the knees and spread the legs, or helped the person spread the legs as much as possible with the knees straight.
19. Placed a waterproof pad under the buttocks.

Procedure—cont'd	S	U	Comments

20. Folded the corner of the bath blanket between the person's legs onto the person's abdomen. ____ ____ _____

21. Wet the washcloths. Squeezed out excess water before using them. ____ ____ _____

22. Applied soap to a washcloth. ____ ____ _____

23. For female perineal care:

     a. Separated the labia. Cleaned downward from front to back with one stroke. ____ ____ _____

     b. Repeated steps 22 and 23a until the area was clean. Used a clean part of the washcloth for each stroke. Used more than one washcloth if needed. ____ ____ _____

     c. Rinsed the perineum with a clean washcloth. Separated the labia. Stroked downward from front to back. Repeated as necessary. Used a clean part of the washcloth for each stroke. Used more than one washcloth if needed. ____ ____ _____

     d. Patted the area dry with the towel. ____ ____ _____

24. For male perineal care:

     a. Retracted the foreskin if the person was uncircumcised. ____ ____ _____

     b. Grasped the penis. ____ ____ _____

     c. Cleaned the tip. Used a circular motion. Started at the urethra and worked outward. Repeated as needed. Used a clean part of the washcloth each time. ____ ____ _____

     d. Rinsed the area with another washcloth. ____ ____ _____

     e. Returned the foreskin to its natural position. ____ ____ _____

     f. Cleaned the shaft of the penis. Used firm downward strokes. Rinsed the area. ____ ____ _____

     g. Helped the person flex his knees and spread his legs. Or helped him spread his legs as much as possible with his knees straight. ____ ____ _____

     h. Cleaned the scrotum. Rinsed well. Observed for redness and irritation in skin folds. ____ ____ _____

     i. Patted dry the penis and scrotum. ____ ____ _____

25. Folded the blanket back between the legs. ____ ____ _____

26. Helped the person lower the legs and turn onto the side away from you. ____ ____ _____

27. Applied soap to a washcloth. ____ ____ _____

28. Cleaned the rectal area with one stroke. For a female, cleaned from the vagina to the anus. ____ ____ _____

29. Repeated steps 27 and 28 until the area was clean. Used a clean part of the washcloth for each stroke. Used more than one washcloth if needed. ____ ____ _____

30. Rinsed the rectal area with a washcloth. For a female, stroked from the vagina to the anus. Repeated as necessary. Used a clean part of the washcloth for each stroke. Used more than one washcloth if needed. ____ ____ _____

31. Patted the area dry with the towel. ____ ____ _____

Continued

Procedure—cont'd

	S	U	Comments
32. Removed the waterproof pad.	___	___	_____
33. Removed and discarded the gloves. Decontaminated hands.	___	___	_____

Post-Procedure

34. Provided for comfort.	___	___	_____
35. Covered the person. Removed the bath blanket.	___	___	_____
36. Lowered the bed to its lowest position.	___	___	_____
37. Raised or lowered bed rails. Followed the care plan.	___	___	_____
38. Placed the signal light within reach.	___	___	_____
39. Emptied and cleaned the wash basin. Wore gloves.	___	___	_____
40. Returned the basin and supplies to their proper place.	___	___	_____
41. Wiped off the overbed table with the paper towels. Discarded the paper towels.	___	___	_____
42. Removed the gloves. Decontaminated hands.	___	___	_____
43. Unscreened the person.	___	___	_____
44. Completed a safety check of the room.	___	___	_____
45. Followed center policy for dirty linen.	___	___	_____
46. Decontaminated hands.	___	___	_____
47. Reported and recorded observations.	___	___	_____

Date of Satisfactory Completion _____ Instructor's Initials _____

Brushing and Combing the Person's Hair

Name: _____   Date: _____

Quality of Life	S	U	Comments
• Knocked before entering the person's room	___	___	_____
• Addressed the person by name	___	___	_____
• Introduced yourself by name and title	___	___	_____

Pre-Procedure

1. Followed Delegation Guidelines. Reviewed Safety Alert.   ___ ___ _____
2. Practiced hand hygiene   ___ ___ _____
3. Identified the person. Checked the ID bracelet against the assignment sheet. Called the person by name.   ___ ___ _____
4. Explained the procedure to the person. Asked the person how to style hair.   ___ ___ _____
5. Collected the following:
   • Comb and brush   ___ ___ _____
   • Bath towel   ___ ___ _____
   • Hair care items as requested   ___ ___ _____
6. Arranged items on the bedside stand.   ___ ___ _____
7. Provided for privacy.   ___ ___ _____

Procedure

8. Lowered the bed rail if used.   ___ ___ _____
9. Helped the person to the chair. The person put on a robe and nonskid footwear. (If the person was in bed, raised the bed for body mechanics. Bed rails were up if used. Lowered the near bed rail. Assisted the person to semi-Fowler's position if allowed.)   ___ ___ _____
10. Placed a towel across the shoulders or across the pillow.   ___ ___ _____
11. Asked the person to remove eyeglasses. Put them in the eyeglass case. Put the case inside the bedside stand.   ___ ___ _____
12. Parted hair into 2 sections. Divided one side into 2 sections. Used the comb   ___ ___ _____
13. Brushed the hair. Started at the scalp and brushed toward the hair ends.   ___ ___ _____
14. Used the comb to divide the other side into sections. Brushed the hair as in step 13.   ___ ___ _____
15. Styled the hair as the person preferred.   ___ ___ _____
16. Removed the towel.   ___ ___ _____
17. Let the person put on the eyeglasses.   ___ ___ _____

Post-Procedure

18. Provided for comfort.   ___ ___ _____
19. Lowered the bed to its lowest position.   ___ ___ _____
20. Raised or lowered bed rails. Followed the care plan.   ___ ___ _____

Continued

Procedure—cont'd

	S	U	Comments
21. Placed the signal light within reach.	____	____	_____
22. Unscreened the person.	____	____	_____
23. Cleaned and returned items to their proper place.	____	____	_____
24. Completed a safety check of the room.	____	____	_____
25. Followed center policy for dirty linen.	____	____	_____
26. Decontaminated hands.	____	____	_____

Date of Satisfactory Completion _____ Instructor's Initials _____

Shampooing the Person's Hair

Name: _____   Date: _____

Quality of Life	**S**	**U**	**Comments**
• Knocked before entering the person's room	___	___	_____
• Addressed the person by name	___	___	_____
• Introduced yourself by name and title	___	___	_____

Pre-Procedure

	S	**U**	**Comments**
1. Followed Delegation Guidelines. Reviewed Safety Alert.	___	___	_____
2. Explained the procedure to the person.	___	___	_____
3. Practiced hand hygiene.	___	___	_____
4. Collected the following:			
• Two bath towels	___	___	_____
• Hand towel or washcloth	___	___	_____
• Shampoo	___	___	_____
• Hair conditioner (if requested)	___	___	_____
• Bath thermometer	___	___	_____
• Pitcher or nozzle (if needed)	___	___	_____
• Shampoo tray (if needed)	___	___	_____
• Basin or pan (if needed)	___	___	_____
• Waterproof pad (if needed)	___	___	_____
• Gloves (if needed)	___	___	_____
• Comb and brush	___	___	_____
• Hair dryer	___	___	_____
5. Arranged items nearby.	___	___	_____
6. Identified the person. Checked the ID bracelet against the assignment sheet. Called the person by name.	___	___	_____
7. Provided for privacy.	___	___	_____
8. Raised the bed for body mechanics for a shampoo in bed. The far bed rail was up if bed rails were used.	___	___	_____

Procedure

	S	**U**	**Comments**
9. Positioned the person for the method you used. Placed the waterproof pad and shampoo tray under the head and shoulders if needed.	___	___	_____
10. Placed a bath towel across the shoulders or across the pillow.	___	___	_____
11. Brushed and combed the hair to remove snarls and tangles.	___	___	_____
12. Raised the bed rail if used.	___	___	_____
13. Obtained water. Tested temperature according to center policy.	___	___	_____
14. Lowered the bed rail if used.	___	___	_____
15. Put on gloves (if needed).	___	___	_____
16. Asked the person to hold a dampened hand towel or washcloth over the eyes. It did not cover the nose and mouth.	___	___	_____
17. Used the pitcher or nozzle to wet the hair.	___	___	_____

Continued

Procedure—cont'd	S	U	Comments
18. Applied a small amount of shampoo.			
19. Worked up a lather with both hands. Started at the hairline. Worked toward the back of the head.			
20. Massaged the scalp with the fingertips. Did not scratch the scalp.			
21. Rinsed the hair.			
22. Repeated steps 18 through 21.			
23. Applied conditioner. Followed directions on the container.			
24. Squeezed water from the person's hair.			
25. Covered hair with a bath towel.			
26. Dried the person's face with a towel.			
27. Helped the person raise the head if appropriate. For the person in bed, raised the head of the bed.			
28. Rubbed the hair and scalp with the towel. Used the second towel if the first was wet.			
29. Combed the hair to remove snarls and tangles.			
30. Dried and styled hair as quickly as possible.			

Post-Procedure

	S	U	Comments
31. Removed and discarded the gloves (if used). Decontaminated hands.			
32. Provided for comfort.			
33. Lowered the bed to its lowest position.			
34. Raised or lowered bed rails. Followed the care plan.			
35. Placed the signal light within reach.			
36. Unscreened the person.			
37. Cleaned and returned equipment to its proper place. Discarded disposable items.			
38. Completed a safety check of the room.			
39. Followed center policy for dirty linen.			
40. Decontaminated hands.			

Date of Satisfactory Completion _____ Instructor's Initials _____

Shaving the Person

Name: _____   Date: _____

Quality of Life	S	U	Comments
• Knocked before entering the person's room	___	___	_____
• Addressed the person by name	___	___	_____
• Introduced yourself by name and title	___	___	_____

Pre-Procedure

	S	U	Comments
1. Followed Delegation Guidelines. Reviewed Safety Alert.	___	___	_____
2. Explained the procedure to the person.	___	___	_____
3. Practiced hand hygiene.	___	___	_____
4. Collected the following:			
• Wash basin	___	___	_____
• Bath towel	___	___	_____
• Hand towel	___	___	_____
• Washcloth	___	___	_____
• Safety razor	___	___	_____
• Mirror	___	___	_____
• Shaving cream, soap, or lotion	___	___	_____
• Shaving brush	___	___	_____
• After-shave lotion (men only)	___	___	_____
• Tissues or paper towels	___	___	_____
• Paper towels	___	___	_____
• Gloves	___	___	_____
5. Arranged paper towels and supplies on the overbed table.	___	___	_____
6. Identified the person. Checked the ID bracelet against the assignment sheet. Called the person by name.	___	___	_____
7. Provided for privacy.	___	___	_____
8. Raised the bed for body mechanics. Bed rails were up if used.	___	___	_____

Procedure

	S	U	Comments
9. Filled the basin with warm water.	___	___	_____
10. Placed the basin on the overbed table.	___	___	_____
11. Lowered the bed rail near you if up.	___	___	_____
12. Assisted the person to semi-Fowler's position if allowed or to the supine position.	___	___	_____
13. Adjusted lighting to clearly see the person's face.	___	___	_____
14. Placed the bath towel over the chest.	___	___	_____
15. Adjusted the overbed table for easy reach.	___	___	_____
16. Tightened the razor blade to the shaver.	___	___	_____
17. Washed the person's face. Did not dry.	___	___	_____
18. Wet the washcloth or towel. Wrung it out.	___	___	_____
19. Applied the washcloth or towel to the face for a few minutes.	___	___	_____

Continued

Procedure—cont'd   S   U   Comments

20. Put on gloves.

21. Applied shaving cream with hands, or used a shaving brush to apply lather.

22. Held the skin taut with one hand.

23. Shaved in the direction of hair growth. Used shorter strokes around the chin and lips.

24. Rinsed the razor often. Wiped it with tissues or paper towels.

25. Applied direct pressure to any bleeding areas.

26. Washed off any remaining shaving cream or soap. Dried with a towel.

27. Applied after-shave lotion if requested.

28. Removed the towel and gloves. Decontaminated hands.

29. Moved the overbed table to the side of the bed.

Post-Procedure

30. Provided for comfort.

31. Placed the signal light within reach.

32. Lowered the bed to its lowest position.

33. Raised or lowered bed rails. Followed the care plan.

34. Cleaned and returned equipment and supplies to their proper place. Discarded disposable items. Wore gloves.

35. Wiped off the overbed table with the paper towels. Discarded the paper towels.

36. Removed the gloves. Decontaminated hands.

37. Positioned the overbed table for the person.

38. Unscreened the person.

39. Completed a safety check of the room.

40. Followed center policy for dirty linen.

41. Decontaminated hands.

42. Reported nicks, cuts, or bleeding to the nurse. Reported and recorded other observations

Date of Satisfactory Completion _____ Instructor's Initials _____

Giving Nail and Foot Care

Name: _____   Date: _____

Quality of Life	S	U	Comments
• Knocked before entering the person's room	___	___	_____
• Addressed the person by name	___	___	_____
• Introduced yourself by name and title	___	___	_____

Pre-Procedure

1. Followed Delegation Guidelines. Reviewed Safety Alert.   ___ ___ _____
2. Explained the procedure to the person.   ___ ___ _____
3. Practiced hand hygiene.   ___ ___ _____
4. Collected the following:
   - Wash basin or whirlpool foot bath   ___ ___ _____
   - Soap   ___ ___ _____
   - Bath thermometer   ___ ___ _____
   - Bath towel   ___ ___ _____
   - Hand towel   ___ ___ _____
   - Washcloth   ___ ___ _____
   - Kidney basin   ___ ___ _____
   - Nail clippers   ___ ___ _____
   - Orange stick   ___ ___ _____
   - Emery board or nail file   ___ ___ _____
   - Lotion for hands   ___ ___ _____
   - Lotion or petrolatum jelly for feet   ___ ___ _____
   - Paper towels   ___ ___ _____
   - Disposable bath mat   ___ ___ _____
   - Gloves   ___ ___ _____
5. Arranged paper towels and other items on the overbed table.   ___ ___ _____
6. Identified the person. Checked the ID bracelet against the assignment sheet. Called the person by name.   ___ ___ _____
7. Provided for privacy.   ___ ___ _____
8. Assisted the person to the bedside chair. Placed the signal light within reach.   ___ ___ _____

Procedure

9. Placed the bath mat under the feet.   ___ ___ _____
10. Filled the wash basin or whirlpool foot bath $2/3$ full with water. The nurse told you what water temperature to use. Measured water temperature with a bath thermometer or tested it by dipping the elbow or inner wrist into the basin.   ___ ___ _____
11. Placed the basin or foot bath on the bath mat.   ___ ___ _____
12. Helped the person put the feet into the basin or foot bath.   ___ ___ _____
13. Adjusted the overbed table in front of the person.   ___ ___ _____

Continued

Procedure—cont'd	S	U	Comments

14. Filled the kidney basin $^2/_3$ full with water. Measured water temperature. _____ _____ _____

15. Placed the kidney basin on the overbed table. _____ _____ _____

16. Placed the person's fingers into the basin. Positioned the arms for comfort. _____ _____ _____

17. Let the fingers soak for 5 to 10 minutes. Let the feet soak for 15 to 20 minutes. Rewarmed water as needed. _____ _____ _____

18. Decontaminated hands. Put on gloves. _____ _____ _____

19. Cleaned under the fingernails with the orange stick. Used a towel to wipe the orange stick after each nail. _____ _____ _____

20. Removed the kidney basin. Dried the hands and between the fingers thoroughly. _____ _____ _____

21. Clipped fingernails straight across with the nail clippers. _____ _____ _____

22. Shaped nails with an emery board or nail file. _____ _____ _____

23. Pushed cuticles back with the orange stick or a washcloth. _____ _____ _____

24. Applied lotion to the hands. _____ _____ _____

25. Moved the overbed table to the side. _____ _____ _____

26. Washed the feet with soap and a washcloth. Washed between the toes. _____ _____ _____

27. Removed the feet from the basin or foot bath. Dried thoroughly, especially between the toes. _____ _____ _____

28. Applied lotion or petrolatum jelly to the tops and soles of the feet. Did not apply between the toes. Warmed lotion before applying it. _____ _____ _____

29. Removed and discarded the gloves. Decontaminated hands. _____ _____ _____

30. Helped the person put on socks and nonskid footwear. _____ _____ _____

Post-Procedure

31. Provided for comfort. _____ _____ _____

32. Placed the signal light within reach. _____ _____ _____

33. Raised or lowered bed rails. Followed the care plan. _____ _____ _____

34. Cleaned and returned equipment and supplies to their proper place. Discarded disposable items. Wore gloves for this step. _____ _____ _____

35. Removed the gloves. Decontaminated hands. _____ _____ _____

36. Unscreened the person. _____ _____ _____

37. Completed a safety check of the room. _____ _____ _____

38. Followed center policy for dirty linen. _____ _____ _____

39. Decontaminated hands. _____ _____ _____

40. Reported and recorded observations. _____ _____ _____

Date of Satisfactory Completion _____ Instructor's Initials _____

Undressing the Person

Name: _____   Date: _____

Quality of Life	**S**	**U**	**Comments**
• Knocked before entering the person's room	___	___	_____
• Addressed the person by name	___	___	_____
• Introduced yourself by name and title	___	___	_____

Pre-Procedure

1. Followed Delegation Guidelines.   ___ ___ _____
2. Explained the procedure to the person.   ___ ___ _____
3. Practiced hand hygiene.   ___ ___ _____
4. Got a bath blanket and clothes as requested by the person.   ___ ___ _____
5. Identified the person. Checked the ID bracelet against the assignment sheet. Called the person by name.   ___ ___ _____
6. Provided for privacy.   ___ ___ _____
7. Raised the bed for body mechanics. Bed rails were up if used.   ___ ___ _____
8. Lowered the bed rail on the person's weak side.   ___ ___ _____
9. Positioned the person supine.   ___ ___ _____
10. Covered the person with the bath blanket. Fanfolded linens to the foot of the bed.   ___ ___ _____

Procedure

11. To remove garments that opened in the back:
    a. Raised the head and shoulders, or turned the person onto the side away from you.   ___ ___ _____
    b. Undid buttons, zippers, ties, or snaps.   ___ ___ _____
    c. Brought the sides of the garment to the sides of the person. If the person was in a side-lying position, tucked the far side under the person. Folded the near side onto the chest.   ___ ___ _____
    d. Positioned the person supine.   ___ ___ _____
    e. Slid the garment off the shoulder on the strong side. Removed it from the arm.   ___ ___ _____
    f. Repeated step 11e for the weak side.   ___ ___ _____
12. To remove garments that opened in the front:
    a. Undid buttons, zippers, snaps, or ties.   ___ ___ _____
    b. Slid the garment off the shoulder and arm on the strong side.   ___ ___ _____
    c. Raised the head and shoulders. Brought the garment over to the weak side. Lowered the head and shoulders.   ___ ___ _____
    d. Removed the garment from the weak side.   ___ ___ _____
    e. If you could not raise the head and shoulders:
       (1) Turned the person toward you. Tucked the removed part under the person.   ___ ___ _____
       (2) Turned the person onto the side away from you.   ___ ___ _____

Continued

Procedure—cont'd   S   U   Comments

    (3) Pulled the side of the garment out from under the person. Made sure the person would not lie on it when supine. _____ _____ _____

    (4) Returned the person to the supine position. _____ _____ _____

    (5) Removed the garment from the weak side. _____ _____ _____

13. To remove pullover garments:

    a. Undid any buttons, zippers, ties, or snaps. _____ _____ _____

    b. Removed the garment from the strong side. _____ _____ _____

    c. Raised the head and shoulders, or turned the person onto the side away from you. Brought the garment up to the person's neck. _____ _____ _____

    d. Removed the garment from the weak side. _____ _____ _____

    e. Brought the garment over the person's head. _____ _____ _____

    f. Positioned the person in the supine position. _____ _____ _____

14. To remove pants or slacks:

    a. Removed footwear. _____ _____ _____

    b. Positioned the person supine. _____ _____ _____

    c. Undid buttons, zippers, ties, snaps, or buckles. _____ _____ _____

    d. Removed the belt. _____ _____ _____

    e. Asked the person to lift the buttocks off the bed. Slid the pants down over the hips and buttocks. Had the person lower the hips and buttocks. _____ _____ _____

    f. If the person could not raise the hips off the bed:

        (1) Turned the person toward you. _____ _____ _____

        (2) Slid the pants off the hip and buttock on the strong side. _____ _____ _____

        (3) Turned the person away from you. _____ _____ _____

        (4) Slid the pants off the hip and buttock on the weak side. _____ _____ _____

    g. Slid the pants down the legs and over the feet. _____ _____ _____

15. Dressed the person. _____ _____ _____

16. Helped the person get out of bed if he or she was to be up. If the person stayed in bed: _____ _____ _____

    a. Covered the person and removed the bath blanket. _____ _____ _____

    b. Provided for comfort. _____ _____ _____

    c. Lowered the bed to its lowest position. _____ _____ _____

    d. Raised or lowered bed rails. Followed the care plan. _____ _____ _____

Post-Procedure

17. Placed the signal light within reach. _____ _____ _____

18. Unscreened the person. _____ _____ _____

19. Completed a safety check of the room. _____ _____ _____

20. Followed center policy for soiled clothing. _____ _____ _____

21. Decontaminated hands. _____ _____ _____

22. Reported and recorded observations. _____ _____ _____

Date of Satisfactory Completion _____   Instructor's Initials _____

Dressing the Person

Name: _____   Date: _____

Quality of Life	S	U	Comments
• Knocked before entering the person's room	___	___	_____
• Addressed the person by name	___	___	_____
• Introduced yourself by name and title	___	___	_____

Pre-Procedure

	S	U	Comments
1. Followed Delegation Guidelines.	___	___	_____
2. Explained the procedure to the person.	___	___	_____
3. Practiced hand hygiene.	___	___	_____
4. Got a bath blanket and clothing requested by the person.	___	___	_____
5. Identified the person. Checked the ID bracelet against the assignment sheet. Called the person by name.	___	___	_____
6. Provided for privacy.	___	___	_____
7. Raised the bed for body mechanics. Bed rails were up if used.	___	___	_____
8. Lowered the bed rail (if up) on the person's strong side.	___	___	_____
9. Undressed the person.	___	___	_____
10. Positioned the person supine.	___	___	_____

Procedure

	S	U	Comments
11. Covered the person with the bath blanket. Fanfolded linens to the foot of the bed.	___	___	_____
12. To put on garments that opened in the back:			
a. Slid the garment onto the arm and shoulder of the weak side.	___	___	_____
b. Slid the garment onto the arm and shoulder of the strong side.	___	___	_____
c. Raised the person's head and shoulders.	___	___	_____
d. Brought the sides to the back.	___	___	_____
e. If the person was in a side-lying position:	___	___	_____
(1) Turned the person toward you.	___	___	_____
(2) Brought one side of the garment to the person's back.	___	___	_____
(3) Turned the person away from you.	___	___	_____
(4) Brought the other side to the person's back.	___	___	_____
f. Fastened buttons, snaps, ties, or zippers.	___	___	_____
g. Positioned the person supine.	___	___	_____
13. To put on garments that opened in the front:			
a. Slid the garment onto the arm and shoulder on the weak side.	___	___	_____
b. Raised the head and shoulders. Brought the side of the garment around to the back. Lowered the person down. Slid the garment onto the arm and shoulder of the strong arm.	___	___	_____
c. If the person could not raise the head and shoulders:			
(1) Turned the person toward you.	___	___	_____
(2) Tuck the garment under the person.	___	___	_____

Continued

Procedure—cont'd

	S	U	Comments
(3) Turned the person away from you.	___	___	_____
(4) Pulled the garment out from under the person.	___	___	_____
(5) Turned the person back to the supine position.	___	___	_____
(6) Slid the garment over the arm and shoulder of the strong arm.	___	___	_____
d. Fastened buttons, snaps, ties, or zippers.	___	___	_____
14. To put on pullover garments:	___	___	_____
a. Positioned the person supine.	___	___	_____
b. Brought the neck of the garment over the head.	___	___	_____
c. Slid the arm and shoulder of the garment onto the weak side.	___	___	_____
d. Raised the person's head and shoulders.	___	___	_____
e. Brought the garment down.	___	___	_____
f. Slid the arm and shoulder of the garment onto the strong side.	___	___	_____
g. If the person could not assume a semi-sitting position:			
(1) Turned the person toward you.	___	___	_____
(2) Tucked the garment under the person.	___	___	_____
(3) Turned the person away from you.	___	___	_____
(4) Pulled the garment out from under the person.	___	___	_____
(5) Positioned the person supine.	___	___	_____
(6) Slid the arm and shoulder of the garment onto the strong side.	___	___	_____
h. Fastened buttons, snaps, ties, or zippers.	___	___	_____
15. To put on pants or slacks:	___	___	_____
a. Slid the pants over the feet and up the legs.	___	___	_____
b. Asked the person to raise the hips and buttocks off the bed.	___	___	_____
c. Brought the pants up over the buttocks and hips.	___	___	_____
d. Asked the person to lower the hips and buttocks.	___	___	_____
e. If the person could not raise the hips and buttocks:			
(1) Turned the person onto the strong side.	___	___	_____
(2) Pulled the pants over the buttock and hip on the weak side.	___	___	_____
(3) Turned the person onto the weak side.	___	___	_____
(4) Pulled the pants over the buttock and hip on the strong side.	___	___	_____
(5) Positioned the person supine.	___	___	_____
f. Fastened buttons, ties, snaps, the zipper, and the belt buckle.	___	___	_____
16. Put socks and footwear on the person.	___	___	_____
17. Helped the person get out of bed. If the person stayed in bed:			
a. Covered the person and removed the bath blanket.	___	___	_____
b. Provided for comfort.	___	___	_____
c. Lowered the bed to its lowest position.	___	___	_____
d. Raised or lowered bed rails. Followed the care plan.	___	___	_____

Post-Procedure

	S	U	Comments
18. Placed the signal light within reach.	_____	_____	_____
19. Unscreened the person.	_____	_____	_____
20. Completed a safety check of the room.	_____	_____	_____
21. Followed center policy for soiled clothing.	_____	_____	_____
22. Decontaminated hands.	_____	_____	_____
23. Reported and recorded observations.	_____	_____	_____

Date of Satisfactory Completion _____ Instructor's Initials _____

Changing the Gown of a Person With an IV

Name: _____   Date: _____

Quality of Life

	S	U	Comments
• Knocked before entering the person's room	___	___	_____
• Addressed the person by name	___	___	_____
• Introduced yourself by name and title	___	___	_____

Pre-Procedure

1. Followed Delegation Guidelines. Reviewed Safety Alert   ___ ___ _____
2. Explained the procedure to the person.   ___ ___ _____
3. Practiced hand hygiene.   ___ ___ _____
4. Got a clean gown and a bath blanket.   ___ ___ _____
5. Identified the person. Checked the ID bracelet against the assignment sheet. Called the person by name.   ___ ___ _____
6. Provided for privacy.   ___ ___ _____
7. Raised the bed for body mechanics. Bed rails were up if used.   ___ ___ _____

Procedure

8. Lowered the bed rail near you if up.   ___ ___ _____
9. Covered the person with a bath blanket. Fan folded linens to the foot of the bed.   ___ ___ _____
10. Untied the gown. Freed parts that the person was lying on.   ___ ___ _____
11. Removed the gown from the arm with no IV.   ___ ___ _____
12. Gathered up the sleeve of the arm with the IV. Slid it over the IV site and tubing. Removed the arm and hand from the sleeve.   ___ ___ _____
13. Kept the sleeve gathered. Slid your arm along the tubing to the bag.   ___ ___ _____
14. Removed the bag from the pole. Slid the bag and tubing through the sleeve. Did not pull on the tubing. Kept the bag above the person.   ___ ___ _____
15. Hung the IV bag on the pole.   ___ ___ _____
16. Gathered the sleeve of the clean gown that would go on the arm with the IV infusion.   ___ ___ _____
17. Removed the bag from the pole. Slipped the sleeve over the bag at the shoulder part of the gown. Hung the bag.   ___ ___ _____
18. Slid the gathered sleeve over the tubing, hand, arm, and IV site. Then slid it onto the shoulder.   ___ ___ _____
19. Put the other side of the gown on the person. Fastened the gown.   ___ ___ _____
20. Covered the person. Removed the bath blanket.   ___ ___ _____

Post-Procedure

21. Provided for comfort.   ___ ___ _____
22. Placed the signal light within reach.   ___ ___ _____
23. Lowered the bed to its lowest position.   ___ ___ _____

Post-Procedure—cont'd

	S	U	Comments
24. Raised or lowered bed rails. Followed the care plan.	_____	_____	_____
25. Unscreened the person.	_____	_____	_____
26. Completed a safety check of the room.	_____	_____	_____
27. Followed center policy for dirty linen.	_____	_____	_____
28. Decontaminated hands.	_____	_____	_____
29. Asked the nurse to check the flow rate.	_____	_____	_____

Date of Satisfactory Completion _____ Instructor's Initials _____

Giving the BedPan

Name: _____   Date: _____

Quality of Life

	S	U	Comments

- Knocked before entering the person's room
- Addressed the person by name
- Introduced yourself by name and title

Pre-Procedure

1. Followed Delegation Guidelines. Reviewed Safety Alert
2. Provided for privacy.
3. Practiced hand hygiene.
4. Put on gloves.
5. Collected the following:
   - Bedpan
   - Bedpan cover
   - Toilet tissue
6. Arranged equipment on the chair or bed.
7. Explained the procedure to the person.

Procedure

8. Warmed and dried the bedpan if necessary.
9. Lowered the bed rail near you if up.
10. Positioned the person supine. Raised the head of the bed slightly.
11. Folded the top linens and gown out of the way. Kept the lower body covered.
12. Asked the person to flex the knees and raise the buttocks by pushing against the mattress with the feet.
13. Slid your hand under the lower back. Helped raise the buttocks.
14. Slid the bedpan under the person.
15. If the person could not assist in getting on the bedpan:
    a. Turned the person onto the side away from you.
    b. Placed the bedpan firmly against the buttocks.
    c. Pushed the bedpan down and toward the person.
    d. Held the bedpan securely. Turned the person onto the back.
    e. Made sure the bedpan was centered under the person.
16. Covered the person.
17. Raised the head of the bed so the person was in a sitting position.
18. Made sure the person was correctly positioned on the bedpan.
19. Raised the bed rail if used.
20. Placed the toilet tissue and signal light within reach.
21. Asked the person to signal when done or when help was needed.

Procedure—cont'd	S	U	Comments
22. Removed the gloves. Decontaminated hands.	___	___	_____
23. Left the room and closed the door.	___	___	_____
24. Returned when the person signaled or checked on the person every 5 minutes. Knocked before entering.	___	___	_____
25. Decontaminated hands. Put on gloves.	___	___	_____
26. Raised the bed for body mechanics. Lowered the bed rail (if used) and the head of the bed.	___	___	_____
27. Asked the person to raise the buttocks. Removed the bedpan, or held the bedpan and turned the person onto the side away from you.	___	___	_____
28. Cleaned the genital area if the person could not do so. Cleaned from front to back with toilet tissue. Used fresh tissue for each wipe. Provided perineal care if needed.	___	___	_____
29. Covered the bedpan. Took it to the bathroom. Lowered the bed and raised the bed rail (if used) before leaving the bedside.	___	___	_____
30. Noted the color, amount, and character of urine or feces.	___	___	_____
31. Emptied the bedpan into the toilet and flushed. Rinsed the bedpan. Poured the rinse into the toilet and flushed. Cleaned the bedpan with disinfectant.	___	___	_____
32. Removed soiled gloves. Practiced hand hygiene and put on clean gloves.	___	___	_____
33. Returned the bedpan and clean cover to the bedside stand.	___	___	_____
34. Helped the person with hand washing.	___	___	_____
35. Removed the gloves. Decontaminated hands.	___	___	_____

Post-Procedure

	S	U	Comments
36. Provided for comfort.	___	___	_____
37. Placed the signal light within reach.	___	___	_____
38. Raised or lowered bed rails. Followed the care plan.	___	___	_____
39. Unscreened the person.	___	___	_____
40. Completed a safety check of the room.	___	___	_____
41. Followed center policy for soiled linen.	___	___	_____
42. Decontaminated hands.	___	___	_____
43. Reported and recorded observations.	___	___	_____

Date of Satisfactory Completion _____ Instructor's Initials _____

Giving the Urinal

Name: _____   Date: _____

Quality of Life	S	U	Comments
• Knocked before entering the person's room	____	____	_____
• Addressed the person by name	____	____	_____
• Introduced yourself by name and title	____	____	_____

Pre-Procedure

	S	U	Comments
1. Followed Delegation Guidelines. Reviewed Safety Alert.	____	____	_____
2. Provided for privacy.	____	____	_____
3. Determined if the man would stand, sit, or lie in bed.	____	____	_____
4. Practiced hand hygiene.	____	____	_____
5. Put on gloves.	____	____	_____

Procedure

	S	U	Comments
6. Gave him the urinal if he was in bed. Reminded him to tilt the bottom down to prevent spills.	____	____	_____
7. If he was going to stand:			
a. Helped him sit on the side of the bed.	____	____	_____
b. Put nonskid footwear on him.	____	____	_____
c. Helped him stand. Provided support if he was unsteady.	____	____	_____
d. Gave him the urinal.	____	____	_____
8. Positioned the urinal if necessary. Positioned his penis in the urinal if he could not do so.	____	____	_____
9. Provided for privacy.	____	____	_____
10. Placed the signal light within reach. Asked him to signal when done or if he needed help.	____	____	_____
11. Removed the gloves. Decontaminated hands.	____	____	_____
12. Left the room and closed the door.	____	____	_____
13. Returned when he signaled or checked on him every 5 minutes. Knocked before entering.	____	____	_____
14. Decontaminated hands. Put on gloves.	____	____	_____
15. Closed the cap on the urinal. Took it to the bathroom.	____	____	_____
16. Noted the color, amount, and character of the urine.	____	____	_____
17. Emptied the urinal into the toilet and flushed. Rinsed the urinal with cold water. Emptied the rinse into the toilet and flushed. Cleaned the urinal with disinfectant.	____	____	_____
18. Returned the urinal to its proper place.	____	____	_____
19. Removed soiled gloves. Practiced hand hygiene and put on clean gloves.	____	____	_____
20. Assisted him with hand washing.	____	____	_____
21. Removed the gloves. Decontaminated hands.	____	____	_____

Post-Procedure

	S	U	Comments
22. Provided for comfort.	___	___	_____
23. Placed the signal light within reach.	___	___	_____
24. Raised or lowered bed rails. Followed the care plan.	___	___	_____
25. Unscreened him.	___	___	_____
26. Completed a safety check of the room.	___	___	_____
27. Followed center policy for soiled linen.	___	___	_____
28. Decontaminated hands.	___	___	_____
29. Reported and recorded observations.	___	___	_____

Date of Satisfactory Completion _____ Instructor's Initials _____

Helping the Person to the Commode

Name: _____   Date: _____

Quality of Life	S	U	Comments
• Knocked before entering the person's room	___	___	_____
• Addressed the person by name	___	___	_____
• Introduced yourself by name and title	___	___	_____

Pre-Procedure

	S	U	Comments
1. Followed Delegation Guidelines. Reviewed Safety Alert.	___	___	_____
2. Explained the procedure to the person.	___	___	_____
3. Provided for privacy.	___	___	_____
4. Practiced hand hygiene.	___	___	_____
5. Put on gloves.	___	___	_____
6. Collected the following:			
• Commode	___	___	_____
• Toilet tissue	___	___	_____
• Bath blanket	___	___	_____
• Transfer belt	___	___	_____

Procedure

	S	U	Comments
7. Brought the commode next to the bed. Removed the chair seat and container lid.	___	___	_____
8. Helped the person sit on the side of the bed.	___	___	_____
9. Helped the person put on a robe and nonskid footwear.	___	___	_____
10. Assisted the person to the commode. Used the transfer belt.	___	___	_____
11. Covered the person with a bath blanket for warmth.	___	___	_____
12. Placed the toilet tissue and signal light within reach.	___	___	_____
13. Asked the person to signal when done or when help was needed. (Stayed with the person if necessary. Provided privacy. Was respectful.)	___	___	_____
14. Removed the gloves. Decontaminated hands.	___	___	_____
15. Left the room. Closed the door.	___	___	_____
16. Returned when the person signaled or checked on the person every 5 minutes. Knocked before entering.	___	___	_____
17. Decontaminated hands. Put on gloves.	___	___	_____
18. Helped the person clean the genital area as needed. Removed the gloves, and practiced hand hygiene.	___	___	_____
19. Helped the person back to bed using the transfer belt. Removed the transfer belt, robe, and footwear. Raised the bed rail if used.	___	___	_____
20. Put on clean gloves. Removed and covered the commode container. Cleaned the commode.	___	___	_____
21. Took the container to the bathroom.	___	___	_____
22. Checked urine and feces for color, amount, and character.	___	___	_____

Procedure—cont'd	S	U	Comments

23. Emptied the container contents into the toilet and flushed. Rinsed the container.Poured the rinse into the toilet and flushed. Cleaned and disinfected the container. ____ ____ _____

24. Returned the container to the commode. Returned other supplies to their proper place. ____ ____ _____

25. Returned the commode to its proper place. ____ ____ _____

26. Removed soiled gloves. Practiced hand hygiene and put on clean gloves. ____ ____ _____

27. Assisted the person with hand washing. ____ ____ _____

28. Removed the gloves. Decontaminated hands. ____ ____ _____

Post-Procedure

29. Provided for comfort. ____ ____ _____

30. Placed the signal light within reach. ____ ____ _____

31. Raised or lowered bed rails. Followed the care plan. ____ ____ _____

32. Unscreened the person. ____ ____ _____

33. Completed a safety check of the room. ____ ____ _____

34. Followed center policy for soiled linen. ____ ____ _____

35. Decontaminated hands. ____ ____ _____

36. Reported and recorded observations. ____ ____ _____

Date of Satisfactory Completion _____   Instructor's Initials _____

Giving Catheter Care

Name: _____   Date: _____

	S	U	Comments

Quality of Life

- Knocked before entering the person's room
- Addressed the person by name
- Introduced yourself by name and title

Pre-Procedure

1. Followed Delegation Guidelines. Reviewed Safety Alert.
2. Explained the procedure to the person.
3. Practiced hand hygiene.
4. Collected the following:
   - Items for perineal care
   - Gloves
   - Bed protector
   - Bath blanket
5. Identified the person. Checked the ID bracelet against the assignment sheet. Called the person by name.
6. Provided for privacy.
7. Raised the bed for body mechanics. Bed rails were up if used.

Procedure

8. Lowered the bed rail near you if up.
9. Decontaminated hands. Put on the gloves.
10. Covered the person with a bath blanket. Fanfolded top linens to the foot of the bed.
11. Draped the person for perineal care.
12. Folded back the bath blanket to expose the genital area.
13. Placed the bed protector under the buttocks. Asked the person to flex the knees and raise the buttocks off the bed.
14. Gave perineal care.
15. Applied soap to a clean, wet washcloth.
16. Separated the labia (female). In an uncircumcised male, retracted the foreskin. Checked for crusts, abnormal drainage, or secretions.
17. Held the catheter near the meatus.
18. Cleaned the catheter from the meatus down the catheter about 4 inches. Cleaned downward, away from the meatus with one stroke. Did not tug or pull on the catheter. Repeated as needed with a clean area of the washcloth. Used a clean washcloth if needed.
19. Rinsed the catheter with a clean washcloth. Rinsed from the meatus down the catheter about 4 inches. Rinsed downward, away from the meatus with 1 stroke. Did not tug or pull on the catheter. Repeated as needed with a clean area of the washcloth. Used a clean washcloth if needed.

Procedure—cont'd　　　　　　S　　U　　**Comments**

20. Secured the catheter. Coiled and secured tubing.
21. Removed the bed protector.
22. Covered the person. Removed the bath blanket.
23. Removed the gloves. Decontaminated hands.

Post-Procedure

24. Provided for comfort.
25. Placed the signal light within reach.
26. Raised or lowered bed rails. Followed the care plan.
27. Lowered the bed to its lowest position.
28. Cleaned and returned equipment to its proper place. Discarded disposable items. Wore gloves for this step.
29. Removed the gloves. Decontaminated hands.
30. Unscreened the person.
31. Completed a safety check of the room.
32. Followed center policy for soiled linen.
33. Decontaminated hands.
34. Reported and recorded observations.

Date of Satisfactory Completion _____ Instructor's Initials _____

Emptying a Urinary Drainage Bag

Name: _____   Date: _____

Quality of Life	S	U	Comments
• Knocked before entering the person's room	___	___	_____
• Addressed the person by name	___	___	_____
• Introduced yourself by name and title	___	___	_____

Pre-Procedure

1. Followed Delegation Guidelines. Reviewed Safety Alert.   ___ ___ _____
2. Collected equipment:
   • Graduate   ___ ___ _____
   • Gloves   ___ ___ _____
   • Paper towels   ___ ___ _____
3. Practiced hand hygiene.   ___ ___ _____
4. Explained the procedure to the person.   ___ ___ _____
5. Identified the person. Checked the ID bracelet against the assignment sheet. Called the person by name.   ___ ___ _____
6. Provided for privacy.   ___ ___ _____

Procedure

7. Put on the gloves.   ___ ___ _____
8. Placed a paper towel on the floor. Placed the graduate on top of it.   ___ ___ _____
9. Positioned the graduate under the collection bag.   ___ ___ _____
10. Opened the clamp on the drain.   ___ ___ _____
11. Let all urine drain into the graduate. Did not let the drain touch the graduate.   ___ ___ _____
12. Closed and positioned the clamp.   ___ ___ _____
13. Measured urine.   ___ ___ _____
14. Removed and discarded the paper towel.   ___ ___ _____
15. Rinsed the graduate. Returned it to its proper place.   ___ ___ _____
16. Removed the gloves. Practiced hand hygiene.   ___ ___ _____
17. Recorded the time and amount on the intake and output (I&O) record.   ___ ___ _____

Post-Procedure

18. Unscreened the person.   ___ ___ _____
19. Completed a safety check of the room.   ___ ___ _____
20. Reported and recorded the amount and other observations.   ___ ___ _____

Date of Satisfactory Completion _____   Instructor's Initials _____

Collecting a Random Urine Specimen

Name: _____   Date: _____

Quality of Life	S	U	Comments
• Knocked before entering the person's room	___	___	_____
• Addressed the person by name	___	___	_____
• Introduced yourself by name and title	___	___	_____

Pre-Procedure

1. Followed Delegation Guidelines. Reviewed Safety Alert.   ___ ___ _____
2. Explained the procedure to the person.   ___ ___ _____
3. Practiced hand hygiene.   ___ ___ _____
4. Collected the following:
   - Voiding receptacle—bedpan and cover, urinal, or specimen pan   ___ ___ _____
   - Specimen container and lid   ___ ___ _____
   - Label   ___ ___ _____
   - Gloves   ___ ___ _____
   - Plastic bag   ___ ___ _____
5. Labeled the container. Put the container and lid in the bathroom.   ___ ___ _____
6. Decontaminated hands.   ___ ___ _____
7. Identified the person. Checked the ID bracelet against the requisition slip. Called the person by name.   ___ ___ _____
8. Provided for privacy.   ___ ___ _____

Procedure

9. Decontaminated hands. Put on the gloves.   ___ ___ _____
10. Asked the person to void into the receptacle. Reminded the person to put toilet tissue into the wastebasket or toilet.   ___ ___ _____
11. Took the receptacle to the bathroom.   ___ ___ _____
12. Poured about 120 ml (4 oz) of urine into the specimen container. Disposed of excess urine.   ___ ___ _____
13. Placed the lid on the specimen container. Put the container in the plastic bag.   ___ ___ _____
14. Cleaned and returned the receptacle to its proper place.   ___ ___ _____
15. Removed gloves, and practiced hand hygiene. Put on clean gloves.   ___ ___ _____
16. Assisted the person with hand washing.   ___ ___ _____
17. Removed gloves, and practiced hand hygiene.   ___ ___ _____

Post-Procedure

18. Provided for comfort.   ___ ___ _____
19. Placed the signal light within reach.   ___ ___ _____
20. Raised or lowered bed rails. Followed the care plan.   ___ ___ _____
21. Unscreened the person.   ___ ___ _____

Continued

Post-Procedure—cont'd

	S	U	Comments
22. Completed a safety check of the room.	____	____	_____
23. Decontaminated hands.	____	____	_____
24. Reported and recorded observations.	____	____	_____
25. Took the specimen and the requisition slip to the storage area.	____	____	_____

Date of Satisfactory Completion _____ Instructor's Initials _____

Collecting a Midstream Specimen

Name: _____   Date: _____

Quality of Life	S	U	Comments
• Knocked before entering the person's room	____	____	_____
• Addressed the person by name	____	____	_____
• Introduced yourself by name and title	____	____	_____

Pre-Procedure

	S	U	Comments
1. Followed Delegation Guidelines. Reviewed Safety Alert.	____	____	_____
2. Explained the procedure to the person.	____	____	_____
3. Practiced hand hygiene.	____	____	_____
4. Collected the following:			
• Midstream specimen kit (with antiseptic solution)	____	____	_____
• Label	____	____	_____
• Disposable gloves	____	____	_____
• Sterile gloves (if not part of the kit)	____	____	_____
• Voiding receptacle—bedpan, urinal, or commode if needed	____	____	_____
• Plastic bag	____	____	_____
• Supplies for perineal care	____	____	_____
5. Labeled the container. Decontaminated hands.	____	____	_____
6. Identified the person. Checked the ID bracelet against the requisition slip. Called the person by name.	____	____	_____
7. Provided for privacy.	____	____	_____

Procedure

	S	U	Comments
8. Provided perineal care. Removed gloves and decontaminated hands.	____	____	_____
9. Opened the sterile kit.	____	____	_____
10. Put on the sterile gloves.	____	____	_____
11. Poured the antiseptic solution over the cotton balls.	____	____	_____
12. Opened the sterile specimen container. Did not touch the inside of the container or lid. Set the lid down so the inside was up.	____	____	_____
13. *For a female:* cleaned the perineum with cotton balls.	____	____	_____
a. Spread the labia with the thumb and index finger. Used the non-dominant hand. (Now this hand could not touch anything sterile.)	____	____	_____
b. Cleaned down the urethral area from front to back. Used a clean cotton ball for each stroke.	____	____	_____
c. Kept the labia separated to collect the urine specimen (steps 16 and 17).	____	____	_____
14. *For a male:* cleaned the penis with cotton balls.	____	____	_____
a. Held the penis with the non-dominant hand.	____	____	_____

Continued

Procedure—cont'd   S   U   Comments

   b. Cleaned the penis starting at the meatus. Used a cotton ball and cleaned in a circular motion. Started at the center and worked outward. ____ ____ _____

   c. Kept holding the penis until the specimen was collected (steps 16 and 17). ____ ____ _____

15. Asked the person to void into the receptacle. ____ ____ _____

16. Passed the specimen container into the stream of urine. Kept the labia separated. ____ ____ _____

17. Collected about 30 to 60 ml of urine (1 to 2 oz). ____ ____ _____

18. Removed the specimen container before the person stopped voiding. ____ ____ _____

19. Released the labia or penis. ____ ____ _____

20. Let the person finish voiding into the receptacle. ____ ____ _____

21. Put the lid on the specimen container. Touched only the outside of the container or lid. ____ ____ _____

22. Wiped the outside of the container. ____ ____ _____

23. Placed the container in a plastic bag. ____ ____ _____

24. Provided toilet tissue after the person was done voiding. ____ ____ _____

25. Took the receptacle to the bathroom. ____ ____ _____

26. Measured urine if intake and output was ordered. Included the amount in the specimen container. ____ ____ _____

27. Cleaned the receptacle and other items. Returned equipment to its proper place. ____ ____ _____

28. Removed soiled gloves. Practiced hand hygiene. ____ ____ _____

29. Put on clean gloves. ____ ____ _____

30. Assisted the person with hand washing ____ ____ _____

31. Removed the gloves. Decontaminated hands. ____ ____ _____

Post-Procedure

32. Follow steps 18 through 25 in procedure: Collecting a Random Urine Specimen. ____ ____ _____

Date of Satisfactory Completion _____ Instructor's Initials _____

Giving a Small-Volume Enema

Name: _____   Date: _____

	S	U	Comments
Quality of Life			
• Knocked before entering the person's room	___	___	_____
• Addressed the person by name	___	___	_____
• Introduced yourself by name and title	___	___	_____

Pre-Procedure

1. Followed Delegation Guidelines. Reviewed Safety Alert.	___	___	_____
2. Explained the procedure to the person.	___	___	_____
3. Practiced hand hygiene.	___	___	_____
4. Collected the following:			
• Small-volume enema	___	___	_____
• Bedpan or commode	___	___	_____
• Waterproof pad	___	___	_____
• Toilet tissue	___	___	_____
• Gloves	___	___	_____
• Robe and nonskid footwear	___	___	_____
• Bath blanket	___	___	_____
5. Identified the person. Checked the ID bracelet against the assignment sheet. Called the person by name.	___	___	_____
6. Provided for privacy.	___	___	_____
7. Raised the bed for body mechanics. Bed rails were up if used.	___	___	_____

Procedure

8. Lowered the bed rail near you if up.	___	___	_____
9. Covered the person with a bath blanket. Fanfolded top linens to the foot of the bed.	___	___	_____
10. Positioned the person in Sims' or a left side-lying position.	___	___	_____
11. Decontaminated hands. Put on the gloves.	___	___	_____
12. Placed the waterproof pad under the buttocks.	___	___	_____
13. Exposed the anal area.	___	___	_____
14. Positioned the bedpan near the person.	___	___	_____
15. Removed the cap from the enema tip.	___	___	_____
16. Separated the buttocks to see the anus.	___	___	_____
17. Asked the person to take a deep breath through the mouth.	___	___	_____
18. Inserted the enema tip 2 inches into the rectum. Did this when the person was exhaling. Inserted the tip gently. Stopped if the person complained of pain, resistance was felt, or bleeding occurred.	___	___	_____
19. Squeezed and rolled the bottle gently. Released pressure on the bottle after the tip was removed from the rectum.	___	___	_____
20. Put the bottle into the box, tip first.	___	___	_____

Continued

Procedure—cont'd	S	U	Comments

21. Helped the person onto the bedpan; raised the head of the bed. Raised or lowered bed rails according to the care plan, or assisted the person to the bathroom or commode. The person wore a robe and nonskid footwear. The bed was in the lowest position.

22. Placed the signal light and toilet tissue within reach. Reminded the person not to flush the toilet.

23. Discarded disposable items.

24. Removed the gloves. Decontaminated hands.

25. Left the room if the person could be left alone.

26. Returned when the person signaled or checked on the person every 5 minutes. Knocked before entering.

27. Decontaminated hands. Lowered the bed rail if up.

28. Put on gloves.

29. Observed enema results for amount, color, consistency, and odor.

30. Helped the person with perineal care.

31. Removed the bed protector.

32. Emptied, cleaned, and disinfected the bedpan or commode. Flushed the toilet after the nurse observed the results.

33. Returned equipment to its proper place.

34. Removed the gloves. Practiced hand hygiene.

35. Assisted the person with hand washing. Wore gloves.

36. Returned top linens. Removed the bath blanket.

Post-Procedure

37. Provided for comfort.

38. Placed the signal light within reach.

39. Lowered the bed to its lowest position.

40. Raised or lowered the bed rails according to the care plan.

41. Unscreened the person.

42. Completed a safety check of the room.

43. Followed center policy for soiled linen and used supplies.

44. Decontaminated hands.

45. Recorded and reported observations.

Date of Satisfactory Completion _____   Instructor's Initials _____

Collecting a Stool Specimen

Name: _____   Date: _____

Quality of Life	S	U	Comments
• Knocked before entering the person's room	___	___	_____
• Addressed the person by name	___	___	_____
• Introduced yourself by name and title	___	___	_____

Pre-Procedure

	S	U	Comments
1. Followed Delegation Guidelines. Reviewed Safety Alert.	___	___	_____
2. Explained the procedure to the person.	___	___	_____
3. Practiced hand hygiene.	___	___	_____
4. Collected the following:			
• Bedpan and cover or commode	___	___	_____
• Urinal for voiding	___	___	_____
• Specimen pan for the toilet or commode	___	___	_____
• Specimen container and lid	___	___	_____
• Tongue blade	___	___	_____
• Disposable bag	___	___	_____
• Gloves	___	___	_____
• Toilet tissue	___	___	_____
• Laboratory requisition slip	___	___	_____
• Plastic bag	___	___	_____
5. Labeled the container. Decontaminated hands.	___	___	_____
6. Identified the person. Checked the ID bracelet with the requisition slip. Called the person by name.	___	___	_____
7. Provided for privacy.	___	___	_____

Procedure

	S	U	Comments
8. Decontaminated hands. Put on gloves.	___	___	_____
9. Asked the person to void. Provided the bedpan, commode, or urinal for voiding if the person did not use the bathroom. Emptied and cleaned the device.	___	___	_____
10. Put the specimen pan on the toilet if the person would use the bathroom. Placed it at the back of the toilet.	___	___	_____
11. Assisted the person onto the bedpan or to the toilet or commode. The person wore a robe and nonskid footwear when up.	___	___	_____
12. Asked the person not to put toilet tissue in the bedpan, commode, or specimen pan. Provided a bag for toilet tissue.	___	___	_____
13. Placed the signal light and toilet tissue within reach. Raised or lowered bed rails. Followed the care plan.	___	___	_____
14. Removed the gloves, and practiced hand hygiene. Left the room.	___	___	_____
15. Returned when the person signaled or checked on the person every 5 minutes. Knocked before entering. Decontaminated hands.	___	___	_____

Continued

Procedure—cont'd

	S	U	Comments
16. Lowered the bed rail near you if up.	___	___	___
17. Put on the gloves. Provided perineal care if needed.	___	___	___
18. Used a tongue blade to take about 2 tablespoons of stool to the specimen container. Took the sample from the middle of a formed stool. If required by center policy, took stool from two different places on the specimen.	___	___	___
19. Put the lid on the specimen container. Did not touch the inside of the lid or container. Placed the container in the plastic bag.	___	___	___
20. Wrapped the tongue blade in toilet tissue.	___	___	___
21. Discarded the tongue blade into the bag.	___	___	___
22. Emptied, cleaned, and disinfected equipment.	___	___	___
23. Removed the gloves. Decontaminated hands.	___	___	___
24. Returned equipment to its proper place.	___	___	___
25. Helped the person with hand washing. Wore gloves.	___	___	___

Post-Procedure

	S	U	Comments
26. Provided for comfort.	___	___	___
27. Placed the signal light within reach.	___	___	___
28. Lowered the bed to its lowest position.	___	___	___
29. Raised or lowered bed rails. Followed the care plan.	___	___	___
30. Unscreened the person.	___	___	___
31. Completed a safety check of the room.	___	___	___
32. Took the specimen and requisition slip to the storage area.	___	___	___
33. Decontaminated hands.	___	___	___
34. Reported and recorded observations.	___	___	___

Date of Satisfactory Completion _____   Instructor's Initials _____

Preparing the Person for a Meal

Name: _____   Date: _____

Quality of Life	S	U	Comments
• Knocked before entering the person's room	___	___	_____
• Addressed the person by name	___	___	_____
• Introduced yourself by name and title	___	___	_____

Pre-Procedure

	S	U	Comments
1. Followed Delegation Guidelines. Reviewed Safety Alert.	___	___	_____
2. Explained to the person that it was mealtime.	___	___	_____
3. Practiced hand hygiene.	___	___	_____
4. Collected the following:			
• Equipment for oral hygiene	___	___	_____
• Bedpan, urinal, commode, or specimen pan and toilet tissue	___	___	_____
• Wash basin	___	___	_____
• Soap	___	___	_____
• Washcloth	___	___	_____
• Towel	___	___	_____
• Gloves	___	___	_____
5. Provided for privacy.	___	___	_____

Procedure

	S	U	Comments
6. Made sure eyeglasses and hearing aids were in place.	___	___	_____
7. Assisted with oral hygiene. Made sure dentures were in place. Decontaminated hands and wore gloves.	___	___	_____
8. Assisted with elimination. Made sure the incontinent person was clean and dry. Wore gloves and practiced hand hygiene.	___	___	_____
9. Assisted the person with hand washing. Wore gloves and decontaminated hands.	___	___	_____
10. Did the following if the person ate in bed:			
a. Raised the head of the bed to a comfortable position.	___	___	_____
b. Cleaned the overbed table. Adjusted it in front of the person.	___	___	_____
c. Placed the signal light within reach.	___	___	_____
d. Unscreened the person.	___	___	_____
11. Did the following if the person sat in a chair:			
a. Positioned the person in a chair or wheelchair.	___	___	_____
b. Removed items from the overbed table. Cleaned the table.	___	___	_____
c. Adjusted the overbed table in front of the person.	___	___	_____
d. Placed the signal light within reach.	___	___	_____
e. Unscreened the person.	___	___	_____
12. Completed a safety check of the room.	___	___	_____
13. Assisted the person to the dining area (if the person ate in the dining area).	___	___	_____

Continued

Post-Procedure

	S	U	Comments
14. Returned to the room. Knocked before entering.	___	___	_____
15. Cleaned and returned equipment to its proper place. Wore gloves.	___	___	_____
16. Straightened the room. Eliminated unpleasant noise, odors, or equipment.	___	___	_____
17. Completed a safety check of the room.	___	___	_____
18. Removed the gloves. Decontaminated hands.	___	___	_____

Date of Satisfactory Completion _____ Instructor's Initials _____

Serving Meal Trays

Name: _____   Date: _____

Quality of Life	S	U	Comments
• Knocked before entering the person's room	___	___	_____
• Addressed the person by name	___	___	_____
• Introduced yourself by name and title	___	___	_____

Pre-Procedure

	S	U	Comments
1. Followed Delegation Guidelines. Reviewed Safety Alert.	___	___	_____
2. Practiced hand hygiene.	___	___	_____

Procedure

	S	U	Comments
3. Made sure the tray was complete. Checked items on the tray with the dietary card. Made sure adaptive equipment was included.	___	___	_____
4. Identified the person. Checked the ID bracelet with the dietary card. Called the person by name.	___	___	_____
5. Placed the tray within the person's reach. Adjusted the overbed table as needed.	___	___	_____
6. Removed food covers. Opened cartons, cut meat, and buttered bread as needed.	___	___	_____
7. Placed the napkin, clothes protector, adaptive equipment, and silverware within reach.	___	___	_____
8. Measured and recorded intake if ordered. Noted the amount and type of foods eaten.	___	___	_____
9. Checked for and removed any food in the mouth. Wore gloves. Decontaminated hands after removing the gloves.	___	___	_____
10. Removed the tray.	___	___	_____
11. Cleaned spills. Changed soiled linen.	___	___	_____
12. Helped the person return to bed if indicated.	___	___	_____

Post-Procedure

	S	U	Comments
13. Assisted the person with oral hygiene and handwashing. Wore gloves.	___	___	_____
14. Removed the gloves. Decontaminated hands.	___	___	_____
15. Provided for comfort.	___	___	_____
16. Placed the signal light within reach.	___	___	_____
17. Raised or lowered bed rails. Followed the care plan.	___	___	_____
18. Completed a safety check of the room.	___	___	_____
19. Followed center policy for soiled linen.	___	___	_____
20. Decontaminated hands.	___	___	_____
21. Reported and recorded observations.	___	___	_____

Date of Satisfactory Completion _____   Instructor's Initials _____

Feeding the Person

Name: _____   Date: _____

Quality of Life	S	U	Comments

- Knocked before entering the person's room   _____ _____ _____
- Addressed the person by name   _____ _____ _____
- Introduced yourself by name and title   _____ _____ _____

Pre-Procedure

1. Followed Delegation Guidelines. Reviewed Safety Alert.   _____ _____ _____
2. Explained the procedure to the person.   _____ _____ _____
3. Practiced hand hygiene.   _____ _____ _____
4. Positioned the person in a sitting position.   _____ _____ _____
5. Got the tray. Placed it on the overbed table or dining table.   _____ _____ _____

Procedure

6. Identified the person. Checked the ID bracelet with the dietary card. Called the person by name.   _____ _____ _____
7. Draped a napkin across the person's chest and underneath the chin.   _____ _____ _____
8. Told the person what foods and fluids were on the tray.   _____ _____ _____
9. Prepared food for eating. Seasoned food as the person preferred and was allowed on the care plan.   _____ _____ _____
10. Served foods in the order the person preferred. Alternated between solid and liquid foods. Used a spoon for safety. Allowed enough time for chewing. Did not rush the person.   _____ _____ _____
11. Used straws for liquids if the person could not drink out of a glass or cup. Had one straw for each liquid. Provided short straws for a weak person.   _____ _____ _____
12. Followed the care plan if the person had dysphagia. Gave thickened liquid with a spoon.   _____ _____ _____
13. Talked with the person in a pleasant manner. Encouraged the person to eat as much as possible.   _____ _____ _____
14. Wiped the person's mouth with a napkin. Discarded the napkin.   _____ _____ _____
15. Noted how much and which foods were eaten.   _____ _____ _____
16. Measured and recorded intake if ordered.   _____ _____ _____
17. Removed the tray.   _____ _____ _____
18. Assisted the person back to his or her room. Practiced hand hygiene and put on gloves.   _____ _____ _____
19. Assisted the person with oral hygiene and hand washing. Provided for privacy. Decontaminated your hands and wore gloves. Decontaminated hands after removing the gloves.   _____ _____ _____

Post-Procedure

	S	U	Comments
20. Provided for comfort.	_____	_____	_____
21. Placed the signal light within reach.	_____	_____	_____
22. Raised or lowered bed rails. Followed the care plan.	_____	_____	_____
23. Completed a safety check of the room.	_____	_____	_____
24. Decontaminated hands.	_____	_____	_____
25. Reported and recorded observations.	_____	_____	_____

Date of Satisfactory Completion _____ Instructor's Initials _____

Applying Elastic Stockings

Name: _____   Date: _____

Quality of Life	S	U	Comments
• Knocked before entering the person's room	___	___	_____
• Addressed the person by name	___	___	_____
• Introduced yourself by name and title	___	___	_____

Pre-Procedure

	S	U	Comments
1. Followed Delegation Guidelines. Reviewed Safety Alert.	___	___	_____
2. Explained the procedure to the person.	___	___	_____
3. Practiced hand hygiene.	___	___	_____
4. Obtained elastic stockings in the correct size and length.	___	___	_____
5. Identified the person. Checked the ID bracelet against the assignment sheet. Called the person by name.	___	___	_____
6. Provided for privacy.	___	___	_____
7. Raised the bed for body mechanics. Bed rails were up if used.	___	___	_____

Procedure

	S	U	Comments
8. Lowered the bed rail near you if up.	___	___	_____
9. Positioned the person supine.	___	___	_____
10. Exposed the legs. Fanfolded top linens toward the thighs.	___	___	_____
11. Turned the stocking inside out down to the heel.	___	___	_____
12. Slipped the foot of the stocking over the toes, foot, and heel.	___	___	_____
13. Grasped the stocking top. Pulled it up the leg. The stocking was even and snug.	___	___	_____
14. Removed twists, creases, or wrinkles.	___	___	_____
15. Repeated steps 11 through 14 for the other leg.	___	___	_____

Post-Procedure

	S	U	Comments
16. Covered the person.	___	___	_____
17. Provided for comfort.	___	___	_____
18. Lowered the bed.	___	___	_____
19. Raised or lowered bed rails. Followed the care plan.	___	___	_____
20. Placed the signal light within reach.	___	___	_____
21. Unscreened the person.	___	___	_____
22. Completed a safety check of the room.	___	___	_____
23. Decontaminated hands.	___	___	_____
24. Reported and recorded observations.	___	___	_____

Date of Satisfactory Completion _____   Instructor's Initials _____

Moving the Person Up in Bed

Name: _____   Date: _____

Quality of Life	S	U	Comments
• Knocked before entering the person's room	___	___	_____
• Addressed the person by name	___	___	_____
• Introduced yourself by name and title	___	___	_____

Pre-Procedure

	S	U	Comments
1. Followed Delegation Guidelines. Reviewed Safety Alert.	___	___	_____
2. Asked a co-worker to assist if needed.	___	___	_____
3. Practiced hand hygiene.	___	___	_____
4. Identified the person. Checked the ID bracelet against the assignment sheet. Called the person by name.	___	___	_____
5. Explained the procedure to the person.	___	___	_____
6. Provided for privacy.	___	___	_____
7. Locked the bed wheels.	___	___	_____
8. Raised the bed for body mechanics. Bed rails were up if used.	___	___	_____

Procedure

	S	U	Comments
9. Lowered the head of the bed to a level appropriate for the person. It was as flat as possible.	___	___	_____
10. Stood on one side of the bed. The co-worker stood on the other side.	___	___	_____
11. Lowered the bed rail near you if up. The co-worker did the same.	___	___	_____
12. Removed pillows as directed by the nurse. Placed a pillow against the headboard if the person could be without it.	___	___	_____
13. Stood with a wide base of support. Pointed the foot near the head of the bed toward the head of the bed. Faced the head of the bed.	___	___	_____
14. Bent your hips and knees. Kept your back straight.	___	___	_____
15. Placed one arm under the person's shoulder and one arm under the thighs. The co-worker did the same. Grasped each other's forearms.	___	___	_____
16. Asked the person to grasp the trapeze if he or she had one.	___	___	_____
17. Had the person flex both knees.	___	___	_____
18. Explained that you would move on the count of "3." The person pushed against the bed with the feet if able.	___	___	_____
19. Moved the person to the head of the bed on the count of "3." Shifted weight from the rear leg to the front leg.	___	___	_____
20. Repeated steps 13 through 19 if necessary.	___	___	_____

Post-Procedure

	S	U	Comments
21. Put a pillow under the person's head and shoulders. Straightened linens.	___	___	_____
22. Provided for comfort. Positioned the person in good alignment.	___	___	_____

Continued

Procedure—cont'd

	S	U	Comments
23. Placed the signal light within reach.	___	___	_____
24. Raised or lowered bed rails. Followed the care plan.	___	___	_____
25. Raised the head of the bed to a level appropriate for the person.	___	___	_____
26. Lowered the bed to its lowest position.	___	___	_____
27. Unscreened the person.	___	___	_____
28. Completed a safety check of the room.	___	___	_____
29. Decontaminated hands.	___	___	_____
30. Reported and recorded observations.	___	___	_____

Date of Satisfactory Completion _____   Instructor's Initials _____

Moving the Person Up in Bed With a Lift Sheet

Name: _____   Date: _____

Quality of Life	S	U	Comments
• Knocked before entering the person's room	____	____	_____
• Addressed the person by name	____	____	_____
• Introduced yourself by name and title	____	____	_____

Pre-Procedure

	S	U	Comments
1. Followed Delegation Guidelines. Reviewed Safety Alert.	____	____	_____
2. Asked a co-worker to help.	____	____	_____
3. Practiced hand hygiene.	____	____	_____
4. Identified the person. Checked the ID bracelet against the assignment sheet. Called the person by name.	____	____	_____
5. Explained the procedure to the person.	____	____	_____
6. Provided for privacy.	____	____	_____
7. Locked the bed wheels.	____	____	_____
8. Raised the bed for body mechanics. Bed rails were up if used.	____	____	_____

Procedure

	S	U	Comments
9. Lowered the head of the bed to a level appropriate for the person. It was as flat as possible.	____	____	_____
10. Stood on one side of the bed. The co-worker stood on the other side.	____	____	_____
11. Lowered the bed rails if up.	____	____	_____
12. Removed pillows as directed by the nurse. Placed a pillow against the headboard if the person could be without it.	____	____	_____
13. Stood with a broad base of support. Pointed the foot near the head of the bed toward the head of the bed. Faced that direction.	____	____	_____
14. Rolled the sides of the lift sheet up close to the person.	____	____	_____
15. Grasped the rolled up lift sheet firmly near the person's shoulders and buttocks. Supported the head.	____	____	_____
16. Bent your hips and knees.	____	____	_____
17. Moved the person up in bed on the count of "3." Shifted weight from the rear leg to the front leg.	____	____	_____
18. Repeat steps 13 through 17 if necessary.	____	____	_____
19. Unrolled the lift sheet.	____	____	_____

Post-Procedure

	S	U	Comments
20. Put a pillow under the person's head and shoulders. Straightened linens.	____	____	_____
21. Provided for comfort. Positioned the person in good alignment.	____	____	_____
22. Placed the signal light within reach.	____	____	_____
23. Raised or lowered bed rails. Followed the care plan.	____	____	_____
24. Raised the head of the bed to a level appropriate for the person.	____	____	_____

Continued

Procedure—cont'd

	S	U	Comments
25. Lowered the bed to its lowest position.	___	___	_____
26. Unscreened the person.	___	___	_____
27. Completed a safety check of the room.	___	___	_____
28. Decontaminated hands.	___	___	_____
29. Reported and recorded observations.	___	___	_____

Date of Satisfactory Completion _____ Instructor's Initials _____

Moving the Person to the Side of the Bed

Name: _____   Date: _____

Quality of Life	S	U	Comments
• Knocked before entering the person's room	___	___	_____
• Addressed the person by name	___	___	_____
• Introduced yourself by name and title	___	___	_____

Pre-Procedure

	S	U	Comments
1. Followed Delegation Guidelines. Reviewed Safety Alerts.	___	___	_____
2. Asked a co-worker to help if using a lift sheet.	___	___	_____
3. Practiced hand hygiene.	___	___	_____
4. Identified the person. Checked the ID bracelet against the assignment sheet. Called the person by name.	___	___	_____
5. Explained the procedure to the person.	___	___	_____
6. Provided for privacy.	___	___	_____
7. Locked the bed wheels.	___	___	_____
8. Raised the bed for body mechanics. Bed rails were up if used.	___	___	_____

Procedure

	S	U	Comments
9. Lowered the head of the bed to a level appropriate for the person. It was as flat as possible. Removed all pillows as directed by the nurse.	___	___	_____
10. Stood on the side of the bed to which you moved the person	___	___	_____
11. Lowered the bed rail near you if bed rails were used.	___	___	_____
12. Stood with the feet about 12 inches apart. One foot was in front of the other. Flexed the knees.	___	___	_____
13. Crossed the person's arms over the person's chest.	___	___	_____
14. *Method 1:* Moving the person in segments:			
a. Placed your arm under the person's neck and shoulders. Grasped the far shoulder.	___	___	_____
b. Placed your other arm under the mid-back.	___	___	_____
c. Moved the upper part of the person's body toward you. Rocked backward and shifted your weight to your rear leg.	___	___	_____
d. Placed one arm under the person's waist and one under the thighs.	___	___	_____
e. Rocked backward to move the lower part of the person toward you.	___	___	_____
f. Repeated the procedure for the legs and feet. Your arms were under the person's thighs and calves.	___	___	_____
15. *Method 2:* Moving the person with a lift sheet:			
a. Rolled the lift sheet up close to the person.	___	___	_____
b. Grasped the rolled up lift sheet near the person's shoulders and hips. The co-worker did the same. Supported the head.	___	___	_____

Continued

Procedure—cont'd   S   U   Comments

   c. Rocked backward on the count of "3," moving the person
       toward you. The co-worker rocked backward slightly and
       then forward toward you while keeping the arms straight.

   d. Unrolled the lift sheet. Removed any wrinkles.

Post-Procedure

16. Provided for comfort.

17. Positioned the person in good alignment. Followed the nurse's
     directions and the care plan.

18. Placed the signal light within reach.

19. Raised or lowered bed rails. Followed the care plan.

20. Lowered the bed to its lowest position.

21. Unscreened the person.

22. Completed a safety check of the room.

23. Decontaminated hands.

24. Reported and recorded observations.

Date of Satisfactory Completion _____ Instructor's Initials _____

Turning and Positioning a Person

Name: _____   Date: _____

Quality of Life	S	U	Comments
• Knocked before entering the person's room	_____	_____	_____
• Addressed the person by name	_____	_____	_____
• Introduced yourself by name and title	_____	_____	_____

Pre-Procedure

	S	U	Comments
1. Followed Delegation Guidelines. Reviewed Safety Alert.	_____	_____	_____
2. Practiced hand hygiene.	_____	_____	_____
3. Identified the person. Checked the ID bracelet against the assignment sheet. Called the person by name.	_____	_____	_____
4. Explained the procedure to the person.	_____	_____	_____
5. Provided for privacy.	_____	_____	_____
6. Locked the bed wheels.	_____	_____	_____
7. Raised the bed for body mechanics. Bed rails were up if used.	_____	_____	_____

Procedure

	S	U	Comments
8. Lowered the head of the bed to a level appropriate for the person. It was as flat as possible.	_____	_____	_____
9. Stood on the side of the bed opposite to where you turned the person. The far bed rail was up if used.	_____	_____	_____
10. Lowered the bed rail near you if up.	_____	_____	_____
11. Moved the person to the side near you.	_____	_____	_____
12. Crossed the person's arms over the person's chest. Crossed the leg near you over the far leg.	_____	_____	_____
13. Turning the person away from you:			
a. Stood with a wide base of support. Flexed your knees.	_____	_____	_____
b. Placed one hand on the person's shoulder. Placed the other on the hip near you.	_____	_____	_____
c. Pushed the person gently toward the other side of the bed. Shifted your weight from rear leg to your front leg.	_____	_____	_____
14. Turning the person toward you:			
a. Raised the bed rail, if used.	_____	_____	_____
b. Went to the other side. Lowered the bed rail if used.	_____	_____	_____
c. Stood with a wide base of support. Flexed your knees.	_____	_____	_____
d. Placed one hand on the person's far shoulder. Placed the other on the far hip.	_____	_____	_____
e. Rolled the person toward you gently.	_____	_____	_____
15. Positioned the person. Followed the nurse's directions and the care plan. The following is common:	_____	_____	_____
a. Placed a pillow under the head and neck.	_____	_____	_____
b. Adjusted the shoulder. The person should not lie on an arm.	_____	_____	_____
c. Placed a small pillow under the upper hand and arm.	_____	_____	_____

Continued

Procedure—cont'd   S   U   **Comments**

   d. Positioned a pillow against the back. ___ ___ _____

   e. Flexed the upper knee. Positioned the upper leg in front of the lower leg. ___ ___ _____

   f. Supported the upper leg and thigh on pillows. ___ ___ _____

Post-Procedure

16. Provided for comfort. ___ ___ _____
17. Placed the signal light within reach. ___ ___ _____
18. Raised or lowered bed rails. Followed the care plan. ___ ___ _____
19. Lowered the bed to its lowest position. ___ ___ _____
20. Unscreened the person. ___ ___ _____
21. Completed a safety check of the room. ___ ___ _____
22. Decontaminated hands. ___ ___ _____
23. Reported and recorded observations. ___ ___ _____

Date of Satisfactory Completion _____ Instructor's Initials _____

Logrolling the Person

Name: _____   Date: _____

Quality of Life	S	U	Comments
• Knocked before entering the person's room	___	___	_____
• Addressed the person by name	___	___	_____
• Introduced yourself by name and title	___	___	_____

Pre-Procedure

	S	U	Comments
1. Followed Delegation Guidelines. Reviewed Safety Alerts.	___	___	_____
2. Asked a co-worker to help.	___	___	_____
3. Practiced hand hygiene.	___	___	_____
4. Identified the person. Checked the ID bracelet against the assignment sheet. Called the person by name.	___	___	_____
5. Explained the procedure to the person.	___	___	_____
6. Provided for privacy.	___	___	_____
7. Locked the bed wheels.	___	___	_____
8. Raised the bed for body mechanics. Bed rails were up if used.	___	___	_____

Procedure

	S	U	Comments
9. Made sure the bed was flat.	___	___	_____
10. Stood on the side opposite to which you turned the person. The co-worker stood on the other side.	___	___	_____
11. Lowered the bed rails if used.	___	___	_____
12. Moved the person as a unit to the side of the bed near you. Used the turning sheet.	___	___	_____
13. Placed the person's arms across the chest. Placed a pillow between the knees.	___	___	_____
14. Raised the bed rail if used.	___	___	_____
15. Went to the other side.	___	___	_____
16. Stood near the shoulders and chest. The co-worker stood near the buttocks and thighs.	___	___	_____
17. Stood with a broad base of support. One foot was in front of the other.	___	___	_____
18. Asked the person to hold his or her body rigid.	___	___	_____
19. Rolled the person toward you or used a turning sheet. Turned the person as a unit.	___	___	_____

Post-Procedure

	S	U	Comments
20. Provided for comfort. Positioned the person in good alignment. Used pillows as directed by the nurse and care plan. (The following is common unless the person has spinal cord involvement.)	___	___	_____
a. One pillow against the back for support.	___	___	_____
b. One pillow under the head and neck if allowed.	___	___	_____

Continued

Post-Procedure—cont'd

	S	U	Comments
c. One pillow or folded bath blanket between the legs.	___	___	_____
d. A small pillow under the arm and hand.	___	___	_____
21. Placed the signal light within reach.	___	___	_____
22. Raised or lowered bed rails. Followed the care plan.	___	___	_____
23. Lowered the bed to its lowest position.	___	___	_____
24. Unscreened the person.	___	___	_____
25. Completed a safety check of the room.	___	___	_____
26. Decontaminated hands.	___	___	_____
27. Reported and recorded observations.	___	___	_____

Date of Satisfactory Completion _____ Instructor's Initials _____

Helping the Person Sit on the Side of the Bed (Dangle)

Name: _____   Date: _____

Quality of Life	S	U	Comments
• Knocked before entering the person's room	___	___	_____
• Addressed the person by name	___	___	_____
• Introduced yourself by name and title	___	___	_____

Pre-Procedure

	S	U	Comments
1. Followed Delegation Guidelines. Reviewed Safety Alert.	___	___	_____
2. Explained the procedure to the person.	___	___	_____
3. Practiced hand hygiene.	___	___	_____
4. Identified the person. Checked the ID bracelet against the assignment sheet. Called the person by name.	___	___	_____
5. Decided what side of the bed to use.	___	___	_____
6. Moved furniture to provide moving space.	___	___	_____
7. Provided for privacy.	___	___	_____
8. Positioned the person in the side-lying position facing you. The person laid on the strong side.	___	___	_____
9. Locked the bed wheels.	___	___	_____
10. Raised the bed for body mechanics. Bed rails were up if used.	___	___	_____

Procedure

	S	U	Comments
11. Raised the head of the bed to a sitting position.	___	___	_____
12. Lowered the bed rail if up.	___	___	_____
13. Stood by the person's hips. Faced the foot of the bed.	___	___	_____
14. Stood with the feet apart. The foot near the head of the bed was in front of the other foot.	___	___	_____
15. Slid one arm under the person's neck and shoulders. Grasped the far shoulder. Placed your other hand over the thighs near the knees.	___	___	_____
16. Pivoted toward the foot of the bed while moving the person's legs and feet over the side of the bed. As the legs went over the edge of the mattress, the trunk was upright.	___	___	_____
17. Asked the person to hold onto the edge of the mattress.	___	___	_____
18. Did not leave the person alone. Provided support if necessary.	___	___	_____
19. Checked the person's condition:			
a. Asked how the person felt. Asked if the person felt dizzy or lightheaded.	___	___	_____
b. Checked pulse and respirations.	___	___	_____
c. Checked for difficulty breathing.	___	___	_____
d. Noted if the skin was pale or bluish in color.	___	___	_____
20. Helped the person lie down if necessary.	___	___	_____
21. Reversed the procedure to return the person to bed.	___	___	_____

Continued

Post-Procedure

	S	U	Comments
22. Lowered the head of the bed after the person returned to bed. Helped him or her move to the center of the bed.	____	____	_____
23. Provided for comfort. Positioned the person in good alignment	____	____	_____
24. Placed the signal light within reach.	____	____	_____
25. Lowered the bed to its lowest position.	____	____	_____
26. Raised or lowered bed rails. Followed the care plan.	____	____	_____
27. Returned furniture to its proper place.	____	____	_____
28. Unscreened the person.	____	____	_____
29. Completed a safety check of the room.	____	____	_____
30. Decontaminated hands.	____	____	_____
31. Reported and recorded observations.	____	____	_____

Date of Satisfactory Completion _____ Instructor's Initials _____

Applying a Transfer Belt

Name: _____   Date: _____

Quality of Life	S	U	Comments

Quality of Life

- Knocked before entering the person's room _____ _____ _____
- Addressed the person by name _____ _____ _____
- Introduced yourself by name and title _____ _____ _____

Procedure

1. Reviewed Safety Alert. _____ _____ _____
2. Practiced hand hygiene. _____ _____ _____
3. Identified the person. Checked the ID bracelet against the assignment sheet. Called the person by name. _____ _____ _____
4. Explained the procedure to the person. _____ _____ _____
5. Provided for privacy. _____ _____ _____
6. Assisted the person to a sitting position. _____ _____ _____
7. Applied the belt around the person's waist over clothing. Did not apply it over bare skin. _____ _____ _____
8. Tightened the belt so it was snug. It did not cause discomfort or impair breathing. You were able to slide 4 fingers (your open, flat hand) under the belt. _____ _____ _____
9. Made sure that a woman's breasts were not caught under the belt. _____ _____ _____
10. Placed the buckle off center in the front or in the back for the person's comfort. The buckle was not over the spine. _____ _____ _____

Date of Satisfactory Completion _____   Instructor's Initials _____

Transferring the Person to a Chair or Wheelchair

Name: _____   Date: _____

Quality of Life	S	U	Comments

- Knocked before entering the person's room   _____ _____ _____
- Addressed the person by name   _____ _____ _____
- Introduced yourself by name and title   _____ _____ _____

Pre-Procedure

1. Followed Delegation Guidelines. Reviewed Safety Alerts.   _____ _____ _____
2. Explained the procedure to the person.   _____ _____ _____
3. Collected the following:
   - Wheelchair or arm chair   _____ _____ _____
   - Bath blanket   _____ _____ _____
   - Lap blanket   _____ _____ _____
   - Robe and nonskid footwear   _____ _____ _____
   - Paper or sheet   _____ _____ _____
   - Transfer belt if needed   _____ _____ _____
   - Seat cushion or positioning device if needed   _____ _____ _____
4. Practiced hand hygiene.   _____ _____ _____
5. Identified the person. Checked the ID bracelet against the assignment sheet. Called the person by name.   _____ _____ _____
6. Provided for privacy.   _____ _____ _____
7. Decided which side of the bed to use. Moved furniture for moving space.   _____ _____ _____

Procedure

8. Placed the chair at the head of the bed. The chair was even with the headboard.   _____ _____ _____
9. Placed a folded bath blanket, cushion, or positioning device on the seat if needed.   _____ _____ _____
10. Locked wheelchair wheels. Raised the footplates. Removed or swung the front rigging out of the way.   _____ _____ _____
11. Lowered the bed to its lowest position. Locked the bed wheels.   _____ _____ _____
12. Fanfolded top linens to the foot of the bed.   _____ _____ _____
13. Placed the paper or sheet under the person's feet. Put footwear on the person.   _____ _____ _____
14. Helped the person sit on the side of the bed. His or her feet touched the floor.   _____ _____ _____
15. Helped the person put on a robe.   _____ _____ _____
16. Applied the transfer belt if needed.   _____ _____ _____
17. *Method 1:* Using a transfer belt:
    a. Stood in front of the person.   _____ _____ _____
    b. Had the person hold onto the mattress.   _____ _____ _____
    c. Made sure the person's feet were flat on the floor.   _____ _____ _____

Procedure—cont'd	**S**	**U**	**Comments**

d. Had the person lean forward.

e. Grasped the transfer belt at each side. Grasped the belt from underneath.

f. Braced your knees against the person's knees. Blocked the person's feet with your feet or used the knee and foot of one leg to block the person's weak foot. Placed the other foot slightly behind you for balance.

g. Asked the person to push down on the mattress and to stand on the count of "3." Pulled the person into a standing position as you straightened your knees.

18. *Method 2:* No transfer belt:

a. Followed steps 17a through 17c.

b. Placed your hands under the person's arms. Your hands were around the person's shoulder blades.

c. Had the person lean forward.

d. Braced your knees against the person's knees. Blocked the person's feet with your feet or used the knee and foot of one leg to block the person's weak foot. Placed your other foot slightly behind you for balance.

e. Asked the person to push down on the mattress and to stand on the count of "3." Pulled the person up into a standing position as you straightened your knees.

19. Supported the person in the standing position. Held the transfer belt or kept the hands around the person's shoulder blades. Continued to block the person's feet and knees with your feet and knees.

20. Turned the person so he or she could grasp the far arm of the chair. The legs touched the edge of the chair.

21. Continued to turn the person until the other armrest was grasped.

22. Lowered the person into the chair as you bent your hips and knees. The person assisted by leaning forward and bending the elbows and knees.

23. Made sure the buttocks were to the back of the seat. Positioned the person in good alignment.

24. Attached the wheelchair front rigging. Positioned the person's feet on the wheelchair footplates.

25. Covered the person's lap and legs with a lap blanket. Kept the blanket off the floor and the wheels.

26. Removed the transfer belt if used.

27. Positioned the chair as the person preferred. Locked the wheelchair wheels or kept them locked according to the care plan.

Post-Procedure

28. Placed the signal light and other needed items within reach.

29. Unscreened the person.

30. Completed a safety check of the room.

31. Decontaminated hands.

32. Reported and recorded observations.

Date of Satisfactory Completion _____   Instructor's Initials _____

Transferring the Person From a Chair or Wheelchair to Bed

Name: _____   Date: _____

	S	U	Comments
Quality of Life			
• Knocked before entering the person's room	___	___	_____
• Addressed the person by name	___	___	_____
• Introduced yourself by name and title	___	___	_____

Pre-Procedure

1. Followed Delegation Guidelines. Reviewed Safety Alerts.	___	___	_____
2. Explained the procedure to the person.	___	___	_____
3. Collected a transfer belt if needed	___	___	_____
4. Practiced hand hygiene.	___	___	_____
5. Identified the person. Checked the ID bracelet against the assignment sheet. Called the person by name.	___	___	_____
6. Provided for privacy.	___	___	_____

Procedure

7. Moved furniture for moving space.	___	___	_____
8. Raised the head of the bed to a sitting position. The bed was in the lowest position.	___	___	_____
9. Moved the signal light so it was on the strong side when the person was in bed.	___	___	_____
10. Positioned the chair or wheelchair so the person's strong side was next to the bed. Had a co-worker help if necessary.	___	___	_____
11. Locked the wheelchair and bed wheels.	___	___	_____
12. Removed and folded the lap blanket.	___	___	_____
13. Removed the person's feet from the footplates. Raised the footplates. Removed or swung the front rigging out of the way.	___	___	_____
14. Applied the transfer belt if needed.	___	___	_____
15. Made sure the person's feet were flat on the floor.	___	___	_____
16. Stood in front of the person.	___	___	_____
17. Asked the person to hold onto the armrests or placed your arms under the person's arms. Your hands were around the shoulder blades.	___	___	_____
18. Had the person lean forward.	___	___	_____
19. Grasped the transfer belt on each side if using it. Grasped underneath the belt.	___	___	_____
20. Braced your knees against the person's knees. Blocked the person's feet with your feet or used the knee and foot of one leg to block the person's weak foot. Placed your other foot slightly behind you for balance.	___	___	_____
21. Asked the person to push down on the armrests on the count of "3." Pulled the person into a standing position as you straightened your knees.	___	___	_____

Procedure—cont'd   S   U   **Comments**

22. Supported the person in the standing position. Held the transfer belt or kept your hands around the person's shoulder blades. Continued to block the person's knees and feet with your knees and feet.

23. Turned the person so he or she could reach the edge of the mattress. The legs touched the mattress.

24. Continued to turn the person until he or she could reach the mattress with both hands.

25. Lowered the person onto the bed as you bent your hips and knees. The person assisted by leaning forward and bending the elbows and knees.

26. Removed the transfer belt.

27. Removed the robe and footwear.

28. Helped the person lie down.

Post-Procedure

29. Provided for comfort. Covered the person as needed.

30. Followed the care plan for use of bed rails.

31. Placed the signal light and other needed items within reach.

32. Arranged furniture to meet the person's needs.

33. Unscreened the person.

34. Completed a safety check of the room.

35. Decontaminated hands.

36. Reported and recorded observations.

Date of Satisfactory Completion _____   Instructor's Initials _____

Transferring the Person Using a Mechanical Lift

Name: _____   Date: _____

Quality of Life	S	U	Comments
• Knocked before entering the person's room			
• Addressed the person by name			
• Introduced yourself by name and title			

Pre-Procedure

	S	U	Comments
1. Followed Delegation Guidelines. Reviewed Safety Alerts.			
2. Asked a co-worker to help.			
3. Explained the procedure to the person.			
4. Collected:			
• Mechanical lift			
• Arm chair or wheelchair			
• Footwear			
• Bath blanket or cushion			
• Lap blanket			
5. Practiced hand hygiene.			
6. Identified the person. Checked the ID bracelet against the assignment sheet. Called the person by name.			
7. Provided for privacy.			

Procedure

	S	U	Comments
8. Raised the bed for body mechanics. Bed rails were up if used.			
9. Lowered the head of the bed to a level appropriate for the person. It was flat as possible.			
10. Stood on one side of the bed. The co-worker stood on the other side.			
11. Lowered the near bed rail.			
12. Centered the sling under the person. Positioned the sling according to the manufacturer's instructions.			
13. Positioned the person in semi-Fowler's position.			
14. Placed the chair at the head of the bed. It was even with the headboard and about 1 foot away from the bed. Placed a folded bath blanket or cushion in the chair.			
15. Locked the bed wheels. Lowered the bed to its lowest position.			
16. Raised the lift so it could be positioned over the person.			
17. Positioned the lift over the person.			
18. Locked the lift wheels in position.			
19. Attached the sling to the swivel bar			
20. Raised the head of the bed to a sitting position.			
21. Crossed the person's arms over the chest. The person held onto the straps or chains but not the swivel bar.			
22. Raised the lift high enough until the person and sling were free of the bed.			

Procedure—cont'd   S   U   Comments

23. Had the co-worker support the person's legs as you moved the lift and person away from the bed.

24. Positioned the lift so that the person's back was toward the chair.

25. Positioned the chair so the person could be lowered into it.

26. Lowered and guided the person into the chair.

27. Lowered the swivel bar to unhook the sling. Left the sling under the person unless otherwise indicated.

28. Put footwear on the person. Positioned the person's feet on wheelchair footplates.

29. Covered the person's lap and legs with a lap blanket. Kept it off the floor and wheels.

30. Positioned the chair as the person preferred. Locked the wheelchair wheels or kept them unlocked according to the care plan.

Post-Procedure

31. Placed the signal light and other needed items within reach.

32. Unscreened the person.

33. Completed a safety check of the room.

34. Decontaminated hands.

35. Reported and recorded observations.

36. Reversed the procedure to return the person to bed.

Date of Satisfactory Completion _____   Instructor's Initials _____

Transferring the Person To and From a Toilet

Name: _____   Date: _____

	S	U	Comments

Quality of Life

- Knocked before entering the person's room _____ _____ _____
- Addressed the person by name _____ _____ _____
- Introduced yourself by name and title _____ _____ _____

Pre-Procedure

1. Followed Delegation Guidelines. Reviewed Safety Alerts. _____ _____ _____
2. Practiced hand hygiene. _____ _____ _____
3. Made sure the person had an elevated toilet seat. The toilet seat and wheelchair were at the same level. _____ _____ _____
4. Checked the grab bars by the toilet. If they were loose, told the nurse. Did not transfer the person to the toilet if the grab bars were not secure. _____ _____ _____

Procedure

5. Had the person wear nonskid footwear. _____ _____ _____
6. Positioned the wheelchair next to the toilet if there was enough room. If not, positioned the wheelchair at a right angle to the toilet. _____ _____ _____
7. Locked the wheelchair wheels. _____ _____ _____
8. Raised the footplates. Removed or swung front rigging out of the way. _____ _____ _____
9. Applied the transfer belt. _____ _____ _____
10. Helped the person unfasten clothing. _____ _____ _____
11. Used the transfer belt to help the person stand and to turn to the toilet. The person used the grab bars to turn to the toilet. _____ _____ _____
12. Supported the person with the transfer belt while he or she lowered clothing, or had the person hold onto the grab bars for support. Lowered the person's pants and undergarments. Or raised the person's skirt or dress and lowered undergarments. _____ _____ _____
13. Used the transfer belt to lower the person onto the toilet seat. _____ _____ _____
14. Removed the transfer belt. _____ _____ _____
15. Told the person you would stay nearby. Reminded the person to use the signal light or call for help when needed. _____ _____ _____
16. Closed the bathroom door to provide for privacy. _____ _____ _____
17. Stayed near the bathroom. Checked on the person every 5 minutes. Completed other tasks in the person's room. _____ _____ _____
18. Knocked on the bathroom door when the person called. _____ _____ _____
19. Helped with wiping, perineal care, flushing, and hand washing as needed. Wore gloves. Removed the gloves and practiced hand hygiene. _____ _____ _____
20. Applied the transfer belt. _____ _____ _____
21. Used the transfer belt to help the person stand. _____ _____ _____
22. Helped the person with clothing. _____ _____ _____

Procedure—cont'd

	S	U	Comments
23. Used the transfer belt to transfer the person to the wheelchair.	_____	_____	_____
24. Made sure the person's buttocks were to the back of the seat. Positioned the person in good alignment.	_____	_____	_____
25. Positioned the person's feet on the footplates.	_____	_____	_____
26. Covered the person's lap and legs with a lap blanket. Kept the blanket off the floor and wheels.	_____	_____	_____
27. Positioned the chair as the person preferred. Locked the wheelchair wheels or kept them unlocked according to the care plan.	_____	_____	_____

Post-Procedure

28. Placed the signal light and other needed items within reach.	_____	_____	_____
29. Unscreened the person.	_____	_____	_____
30. Completed a safety check of the room.	_____	_____	_____
31. Practiced hand hygiene.	_____	_____	_____
32. Reported and recorded observations.	_____	_____	_____

Date of Satisfactory Completion _____ Instructor's Initials _____

Performing Range-of-Motion Exercises

Name: _____   Date: _____

Quality of Life	S	U	Comments

- Knocked before entering the person's room   ____ ____ _____
- Addressed the person by name   ____ ____ _____
- Introduced yourself by name and title   ____ ____ _____

Pre-Procedure

1. Followed Delegation Guidelines. Reviewed Safety Alert.   ____ ____ _____
2. Practiced hand hygiene.   ____ ____ _____
3. Identified the person. Checked the ID bracelet against the assignment sheet. Called the person by name.   ____ ____ _____
4. Explained the procedure to the person.   ____ ____ _____
5. Obtained a bath blanket.   ____ ____ _____
6. Provided for privacy.   ____ ____ _____
7. Raised the bed for body mechanics. Bed rails were up if used.   ____ ____ _____

Procedure

8. Lowered the bed rail near you if up.   ____ ____ _____
9. Positioned the person supine.   ____ ____ _____
10. Covered the person with a bath blanket. Fanfolded top linens to the foot of the bed.   ____ ____ _____
11. Exercised the neck if allowed by the center and if the RN instructed you to do so:
    a. Placed your hands over the person's ears to support the head. Supported the jaws with your fingers.   ____ ____ _____
    b. Flexion—brought the head forward. The chin touched the chest.   ____ ____ _____
    c. Extension—straightened the head.   ____ ____ _____
    d. Hyperextension—brought the head backward until the chin pointed up.   ____ ____ _____
    e. Rotation—turned the head from side to side.   ____ ____ _____
    f. Lateral flexion—moved the head to the right and to the left.   ____ ____ _____
    g. Repeated flexion, extension, hyperextension, rotation, and lateral flexion 5 times—or the number of times stated on the care plan.   ____ ____ _____
12. Exercised the shoulder:
    a. Grasped the wrist with one hand. Grasped the elbow with the other hand.   ____ ____ _____
    b. Flexion—raised the arm straight in front and over the head.   ____ ____ _____
    c. Extension—brought the arm down to the side.   ____ ____ _____
    d. Hyperextension—moved the arm behind the body. (Did this if the person was in a straight-backed chair or was standing.)   ____ ____ _____
    e. Abduction—moved the straight arm away from the side of the body.   ____ ____ _____

Procedure—cont'd	S	U	Comments

    f. Adduction—moved the straight arm to the side of the body.   ____ ____ _____

    g. Internal rotation—bent the elbow. Placed it at the same level as the shoulder. Moved the forearm down toward the body.   ____ ____ _____

    h. External rotation—moved the forearm toward the head.   ____ ____ _____

    i. Repeated flexion, extension, hyperextension, abduction, adduction, and internal and external rotation 5 times—or the number of times stated on the care plan.   ____ ____ _____

13. Exercised the elbow:

    a. Grasped the person's wrist with one hand. Grasped the elbow with the other hand.   ____ ____ _____

    b. Flexion—bent the arm so the same-side shoulder was touched.   ____ ____ _____

    c. Extension—straightened the arm.   ____ ____ _____

    d. Repeated flexion and extension 5 times—or the number of times stated on the care plan.   ____ ____ _____

14. Exercised the forearm:

    a. Pronation—turned the hand so the palm was down.   ____ ____ _____

    b. Supination—turned the hand so the palm was up.   ____ ____ _____

    c. Repeated pronation and supination 5 times—or the number of times stated on the care plan.   ____ ____ _____

15. Exercised the wrist:

    a. Held the wrist with both hands.   ____ ____ _____

    b. Flexion—bent the hand down.   ____ ____ _____

    c. Extension—straightened the hand.   ____ ____ _____

    d. Hyperextension—bent the hand back.   ____ ____ _____

    e. Radial flexion—turned the hand toward the thumb.   ____ ____ _____

    f. Ulnar flexion—turned the hand toward the little finger.   ____ ____ _____

    g. Repeated flexion, extension, hyperextension, and radial and ulnar flexion 5 times—or the number of times stated on the care plan.   ____ ____ _____

16. Exercised the thumb:

    a. Held the person's hand with one hand. Held the thumb with the other hand.   ____ ____ _____

    b. Abduction—moved the thumb out from the inner part of the index finger.   ____ ____ _____

    c. Adduction—moved the thumb back next to the index finger.   ____ ____ _____

    d. Opposition—touched each fingertip with the thumb.   ____ ____ _____

    e. Flexion—bent the thumb into the hand.   ____ ____ _____

    f. Extension—moved the thumb out to the side of the fingers.   ____ ____ _____

    g. Repeated abduction, adduction, opposition, flexion, and extension 5 times—or the number of times stated on the care plan.   ____ ____ _____

17. Exercised the fingers:

    a. Abduction—spread the fingers and the thumb apart.   ____ ____ _____

    b. Adduction—brought the fingers and thumb together.   ____ ____ _____

Continued

Procedure—cont'd

	S	U	Comments

c. Extension—straightened the fingers so the fingers, hand, and arm were straight.

d. Flexion—made a fist.

e. Repeated abduction, adduction, extension, and flexion 5 times—or the number of times stated on the care plan.

18. Exercised the hip:

   a. Supported the leg. Placed one hand under the knee. Placed the other hand under the ankle.

   b. Flexion—raised the leg.

   c. Extension—straightened the leg.

   d. Abduction—moved the leg away from the body.

   e. Adduction—moved the leg toward the other leg.

   f. Internal rotation—turned the leg inward.

   g. External rotation—turned the leg outward.

   h. Repeated flexion, extension, abduction, adduction, and internal and external rotation 5 times—or the number of times stated on the care plan.

19. Exercised the knee:

   a. Supported the knee. Placed one hand under the knee. Placed the other hand under the ankle.

   b. Flexion—bent the leg.

   c. Extension—straightened the leg.

   d. Repeated flexion and extension of the knee 5 times—or the number of times stated on the care plan.

20. Exercised the ankle:

   a. Supported the foot and ankle. Placed one hand under the foot. Placed the other hand under the ankle.

   b. Dorsiflexion—pulled the foot forward. Pushed down on the heel at the same time.

   c. Plantar flexion—turned the foot down, or pointed the toes.

   d. Repeated dorsiflexion and plantar flexion 5 times—or the number of times stated on the care plan.

21. Exercised the foot:

   a. Continued to support the foot and ankle.

   b. Pronation—turned the outside of the foot up and the inside down.

   c. Supination—turned the inside of the foot up and the outside down.

   d. Repeated pronation and supination 5 times—or the number of times stated on the care plan.

22. Exercised the toes:

   a. Flexion—curled the toes.

   b. Extension—straightened the toes.

   c. Abduction—spread the toes apart.

Procedure—cont'd   S   U   Comments

    d. Adduction—pulled the toes together.   _____ _____ _____

    e. Repeated flexion, extension, abduction, and adduction   _____ _____ _____
        5 times—or the number of times stated on the care plan.

23. Covered the leg. Raised the bed rail if used.   _____ _____ _____

24. Went to the other side. Lowered the bed rail near you if up.   _____ _____ _____

25. Repeated steps 12 through 23.   _____ _____ _____

Post-Procedure

26. Provided for comfort.   _____ _____ _____

27. Covered the person. Removed the bath blanket.   _____ _____ _____

28. Raised or lowered bed rails. Followed the care plan.   _____ _____ _____

29. Lowered the bed to its lowest level.   _____ _____ _____

30. Placed the signal light within reach.   _____ _____ _____

31. Unscreened the person.   _____ _____ _____

32. Returned the bath blanket to its proper place.   _____ _____ _____

33. Completed a safety check of the room.   _____ _____ _____

34. Decontaminated hands.   _____ _____ _____

35. Reported and recorded observations.   _____ _____ _____

Date of Satisfactory Completion _____ Instructor's Initials _____

Helping the Person Walk

Name: _____   Date: _____

Quality of Life	S	U	Comments

- Knocked before entering the person's room   _____ _____ _____
- Addressed the person by name   _____ _____ _____
- Introduced yourself by name and title   _____ _____ _____

Pre-Procedure

1. Followed Delegation Guidelines. Reviewed Safety Alert.   _____ _____ _____
2. Explained the procedure to the person.   _____ _____ _____
3. Practiced hand hygiene.   _____ _____ _____
4. Collected the following:
   - Robe and nonskid shoes   _____ _____ _____
   - Paper or sheet to protect bottom linens   _____ _____ _____
   - Gait (transfer) belt   _____ _____ _____
5. Identified the person. Checked the ID bracelet against the assignment sheet. Called the person by name.   _____ _____ _____
6. Provided for privacy.   _____ _____ _____

Procedure

7. Lowered the bed to its lowest position. Locked the bed wheels. Lowered the bed rail if up.   _____ _____ _____
8. Fanfolded top linens to the foot of the bed.   _____ _____ _____
9. Placed the paper or sheet under the person's feet. Put the shoes on the person.   _____ _____ _____
10. Helped the person to dangle.   _____ _____ _____
11. Helped the person put on the robe.   _____ _____ _____
12. Applied the gait belt.   _____ _____ _____
13. Helped the person stand. Grasped the gait belt at each side. Or placed your arms under the person's arms around to the shoulder blades.   _____ _____ _____
14. Stood at the person's side while the person gained balance. Held the belt at the side and back, or had one arm around the back to support the person.   _____ _____ _____
15. Encouraged the person to stand erect with the head up and back straight.   _____ _____ _____
16. Helped the person walk. Walked to the side and slightly behind the person. Provided support with the gait belt, or had one arm around the back to support the person. Encouraged the person to use the handrail on his or her strong side.   _____ _____ _____
17. Encouraged the person to walk normally. (The heel strikes the floor first.)   _____ _____ _____
18. Walked the required distance if the person tolerated the activity. Did not rush the person.   _____ _____ _____
19. Helped the person return to bed.   _____ _____ _____

Procedure—cont'd

	S	U	Comments
20. Lowered the head of the bed. Helped the person to the center of the bed.	_____	_____	_____
21. Removed the shoes. Removed the paper or sheet over the bottom sheet.	_____	_____	_____

Post-Procedure

	S	U	Comments
22. Provided for comfort. Covered the person.	_____	_____	_____
23. Placed the signal light within reach.	_____	_____	_____
24. Raised or lowered bed rails. Followed the care plan.	_____	_____	_____
25. Returned the robe and shoes to their proper place.	_____	_____	_____
26. Unscreened the person.	_____	_____	_____
27. Completed a safety check of the room.	_____	_____	_____
28. Decontaminated hands.	_____	_____	_____
29. Reported and recorded observations.	_____	_____	_____

Date of Satisfactory Completion _____ Instructor's Initials _____

Applying Restraints

Name: _____   Date: _____

Quality of Life	**S**	**U**	**Comments**

- Knocked before entering the person's room   _____ _____ _____
- Addressed the person by name   _____ _____ _____
- Introduced yourself by name and title   _____ _____ _____

Pre-Procedure

1. Followed Delegation Guidelines. Reviewed Safety Alert.   _____ _____ _____
2. Collected the following as instructed by the nurse:
   - Correct type and size of restraints   _____ _____ _____
   - Padding for bony areas   _____ _____ _____
   - Bed rail pads or gap protectors   _____ _____ _____
3. Practiced hand hygiene.   _____ _____ _____
4. Identified the person. Checked the ID bracelet against the
   assignment sheet. Called the person by name.   _____ _____ _____
5. Explained the procedure to the person.   _____ _____ _____
6. Provided for privacy.   _____ _____ _____

Procedure

7. Made sure the person was comfortable and in good alignment.   _____ _____ _____
8. Put the bed rail pads or gap protectors on the bed if the person
   was in bed, if needed. Followed the manufacturer's instructions. _____ _____ _____
9. Padded bony areas according to the nurse's instructions.   _____ _____ _____
10. Read the manufacturer's instructions. Noted the front and back
    of the restraint.   _____ _____ _____
11. For wrist restraints:
    a. Applied the restraint following the manufacturer's instruc-
       tions. Placed the soft part toward the skin.   _____ _____ _____
    b. Secured the restraint so it was snug but not tight. Made sure
       you could slide one or two fingers under the restraint. Fol-
       lowed the manufacturer's instructions.   _____ _____ _____
    c. Tied the straps to the movable part of the bed frame out of
       the person's reach. Used a center-approved tie. Left 1 to
       2 inches of slack in the straps.   _____ _____ _____
    d. Repeated steps 11a, 11b, and 11c for the other wrist.   _____ _____ _____
12. For mitt restraints:
    a. Made sure the person's hands were clean and dry.   _____ _____ _____
    b. Applied the mitt restraint. Followed the manufacturer's
       instructions.   _____ _____ _____
    c. Tied the straps to the movable part of the bed frame. Used a
       center-approved tie. Left 1 to 2 inches of slack in the straps.

Procedure—cont'd	**S**	**U**	**Comments**

    d. Made sure the restraint was snug. Slid one or two fingers between the restraint and the wrist. Followed the manufacturer's instructions. Adjusted the straps if it was too loose or too tight. Checked for snugness again.

    e. Repeated steps 12b, 12c, and 12d for the other hand.

13. For a belt restraint:

    a. Assisted the person to a sitting position.

    b. Applied the restraint with your free hand. Followed the manufacturer's instructions.

    c. Removed wrinkles or creases from the front and back of the restraint.

    d. Brought the ties through the slots in the belt.

    e. Helped the person lie down if he or she was in bed.

    f. Made sure the person was comfortable and in good alignment.

    g. Secured the straps to the movable part of the bed frame out of the person's reach or to the chair or wheelchair. Used a center-approved tie. Left 1 to 2 inches of slack in the straps.

14. For a vest restraint:

    a. Assisted the person to a sitting position.

    b. Applied the restraint with your free hand. Followed the manufacturer's instructions. The V part of the vest crossed in front.

    c. Made sure the vest was free of wrinkles in the front and back.

    d. Helped the person lie down if he or she was in bed.

    e. Brought the straps through the slots.

    f. Made sure the person was comfortable and in good alignment.

    g. Secured the straps to the chair or to the movable part of the bed frame. If secured to the bed frame, the straps were secured at waist level out of the person's reach. Used a center-approved tie. Left 1 to 2 inches of slack in the straps.

    h. Made sure the vest was snug. Slid an open hand between the restraint and the person. Adjusted the restraint if it was too loose or too tight. Checked for snugness again.

15. For a jacket restraint:

    a. Assisted the person to a sitting position.

    b. Applied the restraint with your free hand. Followed the manufacturer's instructions. The jacket opening was in back.

    c. Closed the back with the zipper, ties, or hook and loop closures.

    d. Made sure the side seams were under the arms. Removed any wrinkles in the front and back.

    e. Helped the person lie down if he or she was in bed.

    f. Made sure the person was comfortable and in good alignment.

Continued

Procedure—cont'd   S   U   Comments

g. Secured the straps to the chair or to the movable part of the bed frame. If secured to the bed frame, the straps were secured at waist level out of the person's reach. Used a center-approved knot. Left 1 to 2 inches of slack in the straps. _____ _____ _____

h. Made sure the jacket was snug. Slid an open hand between the restraint and the person. Adjusted the restraint if it was too loose or too tight. Checked for snugness again. _____ _____ _____

Post-Procedure

16. Positioned the person as the nurse directed. Provided for comfort. _____ _____ _____

17. Placed the signal light within the person's reach. _____ _____ _____

18. Raised or lowered bed rails. Followed the care plan and the manufacturer's instructions for the restraint. _____ _____ _____

19. Unscreened the person. _____ _____ _____

20. Completed a safety check of the room. _____ _____ _____

21. Decontaminated hands. _____ _____ _____

22. Checked the person and the restraints at least every 15 minutes. Reported and recorded observations. _____ _____ _____

   a. For wrist and mitt restraints: checked the pulse, color, and temperature of the restrained parts. _____ _____ _____

   b. For vest, jacket, and belt restraints: checked the person's breathing. Called the nurse at once if the person was not breathing or was having difficulty breathing. Made sure the restraint was properly positioned in the front and back. _____ _____ _____

23. Did the following at least every 2 hours:

   • Removed the restraint. _____ _____ _____

   • Repositioned the person. _____ _____ _____

   • Met food, fluid, hygiene, and elimination needs. _____ _____ _____

   • Gave skin care. _____ _____ _____

   • Performed range-of-motion exercises or ambulated the person. Followed the care plan. _____ _____ _____

   • Provided for comfort. _____ _____ _____

   • Reapplied the restraints. _____ _____ _____

24. Completed a safety check of the room. _____ _____ _____

25. Reported and recorded observations and the care given. _____ _____ _____

Date of Satisfactory Completion _____ Instructor's Initials _____